Plant Based Diet Guide Book:

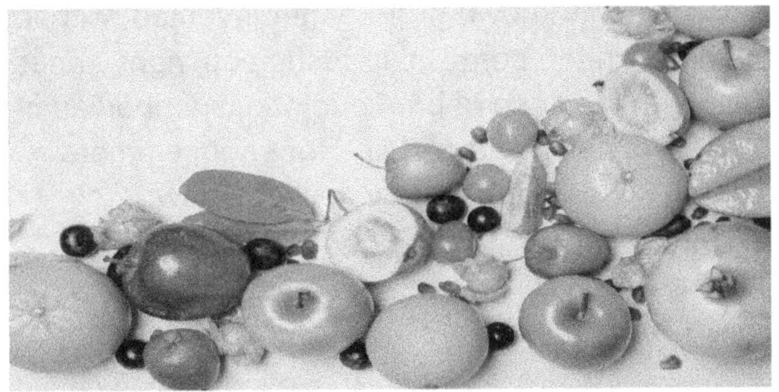

Secrets to Good Health and Wellness.

by

Andrea Rich

Table of Content

Part I: Foundations of a Plant-Based Diet

Chapter 1: What is a Plant-Based Diet?

Chapter 2: Nutritional Science Behind Plant-Based Diets

Chapter 3: Transitioning to a Plant-Based Lifestyle

INTRODUCTION

Welcome to the fascinating world of plant-based nutrition, where the bounty of nature unveils the secret to vibrant health and wellness. In this exploration, we delve deep into the essence of plant-based diets, understanding their profound impact on our well-being and the evolutionary journey that has led us to embrace this transformative lifestyle.

Understanding Plant-Based Diet: At the heart of our journey lies the comprehension of plant-based diets—a lifestyle centered around the nourishment drawn from the rich tapestry of plant-derived foods. It's not merely a diet but a philosophy, an approach that reveres the healing power of nature's offerings. Plant-based eating involves savoring a colorful palette of fruits, vegetables, legumes, whole grains, nuts, and seeds—a symphony of nutrients that nourish our bodies and invigorate our health.

The importance of nutrition in health: Nutrition forms the cornerstone of our well-being, influencing every aspect of our physical and mental health. As we navigate the intricacies of plant-based nutrition, we unveil the significance of consuming a diverse array of vitamins, minerals, phytonutrients, and antioxidants present abundantly in plant-derived foods. Understanding how these nutrients synergize to fuel our bodies is key to unlocking the path to optimal health and vitality.

Evolution of Plant-Based Diets: The journey towards embracing plant-based diets is deeply woven into the fabric of human evolution. Across civilizations and centuries, humans have harmonized with the abundance of nature, relying on plant foods for sustenance and vitality. From ancient civilizations to contemporary societies, the evolution of plant-based diets reflects our innate connection with the earth and the wisdom inherent in consuming whole, unprocessed foods.

Benefits of Adopting a Plant-Based Lifestyle: Embracing a plant-based lifestyle isn't just a dietary shift; it's a profound transformation that reaps a multitude of benefits. From bolstering cardiovascular health, managing weight, enhancing gut health, to fostering mental well-being—the advantages of adopting a plant-based lifestyle are far-reaching. Moreover, this lifestyle choice extends beyond personal health, contributing significantly to the sustainability of our planet by reducing environmental impact and fostering a greener future.

As we embark on this illuminating expedition through the world of plant-based diets, this book aims to serve as your guide—an ally in unraveling the mysteries of nutrition, health, and well-being. Join us as we uncover the magic of plant-based nutrition and unlock the secret to a life brimming with vitality, energy, and wellness.

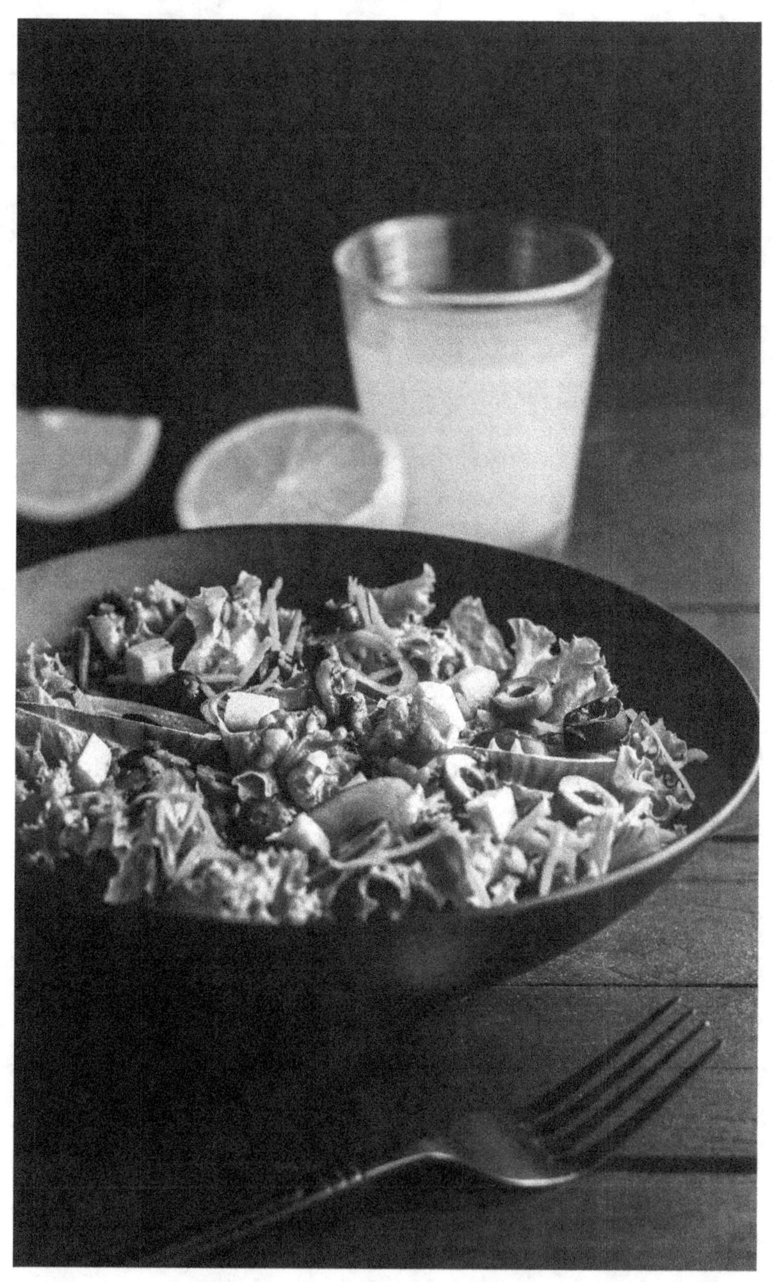

Part I
Foundations of a Plant-Based Diet.

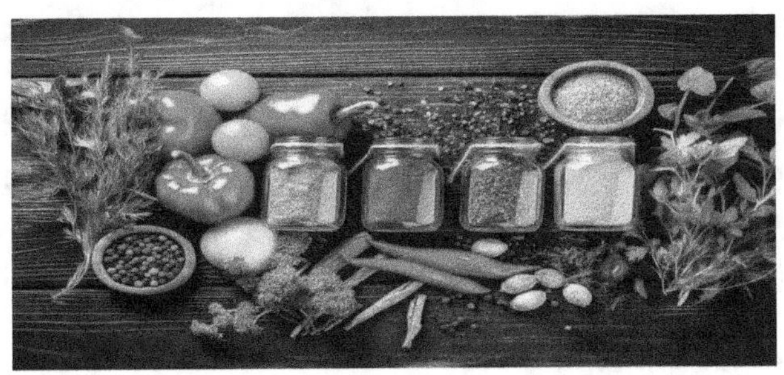

CHAPTER ONE
What is a Plant-Based Diet?

Introduction to Plant-Based Diet

In a world brimming with dietary choices, the concept of a plant-based diet emerges as a beacon of health, vitality, and ethical consumption. It transcends the confines of a mere diet; it embodies a philosophy, a way of life that celebrates the nourishing abundance of nature while fostering holistic well-being for both individuals and the planet.

Embracing the Plant-Based Lifestyle

A plant-based diet revolves around the fundamental principle of centering meals primarily on nutrient-dense, plant-derived foods. It goes beyond the reduction of animal-based products; it's an affirmative choice to savor the vibrancy and wholesomeness present in an array of fruits, vegetables, whole grains, legumes, nuts, seeds, and plant-based oils. This dietary framework celebrates the bountiful gifts of the earth while aligning with the ethical considerations of compassionate eating.

The Philosophical Core

At its core, a plant-based diet resonates with values of environmental stewardship, health consciousness, and ethical treatment of animals. It acknowledges the profound interconnectedness between dietary choices and their impact not only on personal health but also on global sustainability. Choosing a plant-based lifestyle becomes an assertion—a commitment to nurturing personal well-being while participating in the collective responsibility of safeguarding the planet's ecological balance.

Unveiling the Healthful Potentials

Plant-based eating stands as a fountain of health, offering an array of benefits that resonate throughout the human body. Embracing this dietary path has been correlated with reducing the risk of chronic diseases such as cardiovascular ailments, diabetes, and certain cancers. The abundance of fiber, vitamins, minerals, and phytonutrients present in plant foods fortifies the body's defenses, bolsters immunity, and fosters longevity.

Beyond Nutrition: A Holistic Wellness Approach

A plant-based diet transcends the physical realm, extending its influence to mental clarity, emotional balance, and spiritual well-being. The nourishment derived from plant-centric eating patterns isn't merely about the nutrients on the plate; it encompasses a holistic approach to life, promoting mindfulness, vitality, and a profound connection with the environment.

The Journey Ahead

As we embark on this enriching expedition into the realm of plant-based diets, this exploration stands as an invitation—a beckoning call to embrace a lifestyle that not only nourishes our bodies but also champions the welfare of our planet.

Through this journey, we aim to unravel the secrets, dispel myths, and ignite the passion for a life brimming with vitality, health, and ethical harmony.

Join us as we unravel the mysteries, embrace the flavors, and embark on a transformative odyssey through the captivating world of plant-based nutrition—a journey toward vibrant health and holistic well-being.

Defining Plant-Based Diet.

A plant-based diet is a dietary approach centered predominantly on foods sourced from plants. It revolves around consuming a rich variety of fruits, vegetables, whole grains, legumes, nuts, seeds, and plant-derived oils. Unlike strict vegan or vegetarian diets, a plant-based diet accommodates flexibility, allowing individuals to incorporate plant foods while occasionally including small portions of animal-derived products.

At its core, a plant-based diet prioritizes whole, minimally processed foods, harnessing the nutritional bounty present in natural, plant-derived sources. It promotes the consumption of nutrient-dense meals while limiting or eliminating highly processed foods, refined sugars, and excessive fats often associated with animal-based products.

The emphasis on plant-based eating isn't solely about dietary choices; it embodies a lifestyle promoting health, sustainability, and ethical considerations. It acknowledges the positive impact of consuming a wide array of plant-derived nutrients, including vitamins, minerals, antioxidants, and fiber, which collectively contribute to improved overall health and reduced risk of chronic diseases.

This dietary approach isn't confined to specific rules or rigid structures but invites individuals to explore and integrate more plant-derived foods into their daily meals. Whether one adopts a fully plant-based lifestyle or incorporates plant-based meals into their diet intermittently, the underlying philosophy of prioritizing plant-derived foods remains the cornerstone of this approach.

In essence, a plant-based diet celebrates the diverse array of natural, whole foods, harnessing their nutritional potency to promote well-being, environmental sustainability, and a harmonious relationship with the planet.

Approaches to Plant-Based Diets

Embracing a plant-based dietary lifestyle offers a spectrum of choices, accommodating various preferences and needs. Understanding the diverse approaches within plant-based eating helps individuals tailor their dietary patterns to align with their health goals, ethical considerations, and personal beliefs.

1. Veganism

Definition: Veganism represents the most stringent form of plant-based eating, excluding all animal-derived products. This dietary lifestyle abstains from meat, poultry, fish, dairy, eggs, honey, and any other animal-based ingredients.

Emphasis: Vegan diets prioritize whole plant foods, encompassing fruits, vegetables, grains, legumes, nuts, seeds, and plant-based oils. The emphasis lies on cruelty-free consumption, ethical considerations for animals, and environmental sustainability.

2. Vegetarianism

Definition: Vegetarian diets abstain from meat, poultry, and fish but may include dairy products and eggs.

Variants:
- Lacto-Ovo Vegetarian: Includes dairy and eggs while avoiding meat, fish, and poultry.

- Lacto-Vegetarian: Includes dairy but excludes eggs, meat, fish, and poultry.

- Ovo-Vegetarian:Includes eggs but excludes dairy, meat, fish, and poultry.

Emphasis: Vegetarian diets center around plant foods, similar to veganism, but provide flexibility by incorporating dairy or eggs, catering to diverse dietary preferences and cultural backgrounds.

3. Flexitarian or Semi-Vegetarian

Definition: Flexitarian diets allow occasional consumption of animal-derived products without excluding them entirely. These diets are primarily plant-based but allow for limited intake of meat, fish, or poultry on occasion.

Emphasis: Flexitarian diets encourage a plant-centric approach while allowing flexibility for occasional animal product consumption. The focus remains on plant-derived foods, promoting health benefits associated with plant-based eating while offering a less restrictive dietary pattern.

4. Pescatarian

Definition: Pescatarian diets abstain from meat and poultry but include fish and seafood.

Emphasis: Pescatarian diets lean heavily towards plant foods but incorporate fish and seafood for added variety and nutrient sources while avoiding other animal meats.

5. Whole Food Plant-Based (WFPB) Diet

Definition: Whole Food Plant-Based diets emphasize whole, minimally processed plant foods while excluding or minimizing refined products, added sugars, and oils.

Emphasis: WFPB diets focus on consuming whole plant foods in their unprocessed state, prioritizing fruits, vegetables, whole grains, legumes, nuts, and seeds. The emphasis is on nutritionally dense foods, minimizing or eliminating processed items for optimal health benefits.

6. Raw Vegan or Raw Food Diet

Definition: Raw vegan diets solely consist of uncooked, unprocessed plant foods, emphasizing raw fruits, vegetables, nuts, seeds, and sprouted grains.

Emphasis: Raw vegan diets underscore the consumption of raw and unprocessed plant-derived foods, believed to preserve nutrients and enzymes, promoting health and vitality.

7. Plant-Based Ketogenic Diet

Definition: Plant-Based Ketogenic diets adapt the principles of a ketogenic diet (high-fat, moderate-protein, low-carb) while exclusively deriving fats and proteins from plant sources.

Emphasis: This diet combines a ketogenic approach with plant-derived fats and proteins, focusing on low-carb, high-fat foods while excluding animal-derived products.

8. Mediterranean Diet

Definition: The Mediterranean diet predominantly comprises plant-based foods, such as fruits, vegetables, whole grains, legumes, nuts, and seeds, with occasional fish, dairy, and poultry.

Emphasis: While not strictly plant-based, the Mediterranean diet showcases a predominantly plant-centric approach, emphasizing the consumption of heart-healthy plant foods while allowing moderate intake of animal products, primarily fish and dairy.

Navigating the Spectrum

Understanding the varied approaches within plant-based diets offers individuals the flexibility to choose a dietary path that aligns with their preferences, health objectives, cultural backgrounds, and ethical considerations. Each approach presents unique advantages while emphasizing the central theme of prioritizing plant-derived foods for optimal health, environmental sustainability, and ethical consciousness.

Exploring Plant-Based Food Groups

1. Fruits

Nutritional Value: Fruits offer an abundance of vitamins, particularly vitamin C, essential for immune function, skin health, and antioxidant protection. They are rich in dietary fiber, aiding in digestion and promoting satiety. Moreover, fruits contain various antioxidants and phytochemicals, contributing to overall health and disease prevention.

Variety and Benefits: Incorporating a diverse range of fruits—berries, citrus fruits, tropical fruits, and more—ensures a broad spectrum of nutrients. These diverse choices provide different antioxidants, vitamins, and minerals crucial for a well-rounded diet. Each fruit type brings unique health benefits, from supporting heart health to enhancing cognitive function.

2. Vegetables

Nutritional Value: Vegetables are nutritional powerhouses, offering vitamins (such as A, K, and folate), minerals (like potassium, magnesium), dietary fiber, and a myriad of antioxidants. They contribute to maintaining healthy blood pressure, supporting bone health, and reducing the risk of chronic diseases like diabetes and certain cancers.

Variety and Benefits: Including an assortment of vegetables—leafy greens, cruciferous vegetables, root vegetables, and colorful veggies—provides a diverse array of nutrients. Different vegetables offer distinct health benefits, from improving vision and skin health to aiding in detoxification and supporting immune function.

3. Whole Grains

Nutritional Value: Whole grains, such as quinoa, brown rice, oats, barley, and whole wheat, are rich in fiber, vitamins (B-complex vitamins), minerals (iron, magnesium), and antioxidants. They support digestive health, regulate blood sugar levels, and reduce the risk of heart disease.

Variety and Benefits:
Consuming a variety of whole grains ensures a balanced intake of nutrients. Incorporating different grains into meals offers diverse textures, flavors, and nutritional profiles. Whole grains are beneficial for sustained energy levels, weight management, and reducing the risk of chronic illnesses.

4. Legumes

Nutritional Value:
Legumes—beans, lentils, chickpeas, and peas—are excellent sources of plant-based protein, fiber, iron, folate, potassium, and antioxidants. They support muscle growth, aid in digestion, regulate blood sugar, and contribute to heart health.

Variety and Benefits:
Including various legumes in the diet offers a wide range of nutrients and health benefits. Different legumes provide essential amino acids, making them valuable sources of protein in plant-based diets. They are versatile ingredients, adaptable to various cuisines, and contribute to a well-balanced diet.

5. Nuts and Seeds

Nutritional Value: Nuts and seeds are packed with healthy fats (omega-3 fatty acids), protein, fiber, vitamins (E, B-complex vitamins), minerals (magnesium, zinc), and antioxidants. They support brain health, cardiovascular health, and overall well-being.

Variety and Benefits: Incorporating a variety of nuts and seeds—almonds, walnuts, chia seeds, flaxseeds, pumpkin seeds—provides a mix of nutrients. They offer heart-healthy fats, essential minerals, and antioxidants beneficial for reducing inflammation, supporting brain function, and managing cholesterol levels.

6. Plant-Based Oils

Nutritional Value: Plant-based oils like olive oil, avocado oil, and flaxseed oil contain healthy fats, particularly monounsaturated and polyunsaturated fats, along with vitamin E and antioxidants. They support heart health, reduce inflammation, and aid in nutrient absorption.

Variety and Benefits: Including different plant-based oils in cooking and meal preparations provides a source of healthy fats. Choosing oils rich in monounsaturated and polyunsaturated fats supports a balanced lipid profile, benefiting heart health and overall well-being.

Understanding and incorporating these plant-based food groups into one's diet in a balanced and varied manner can significantly contribute to overall health, vitality, and disease prevention in a plant-centric lifestyle.

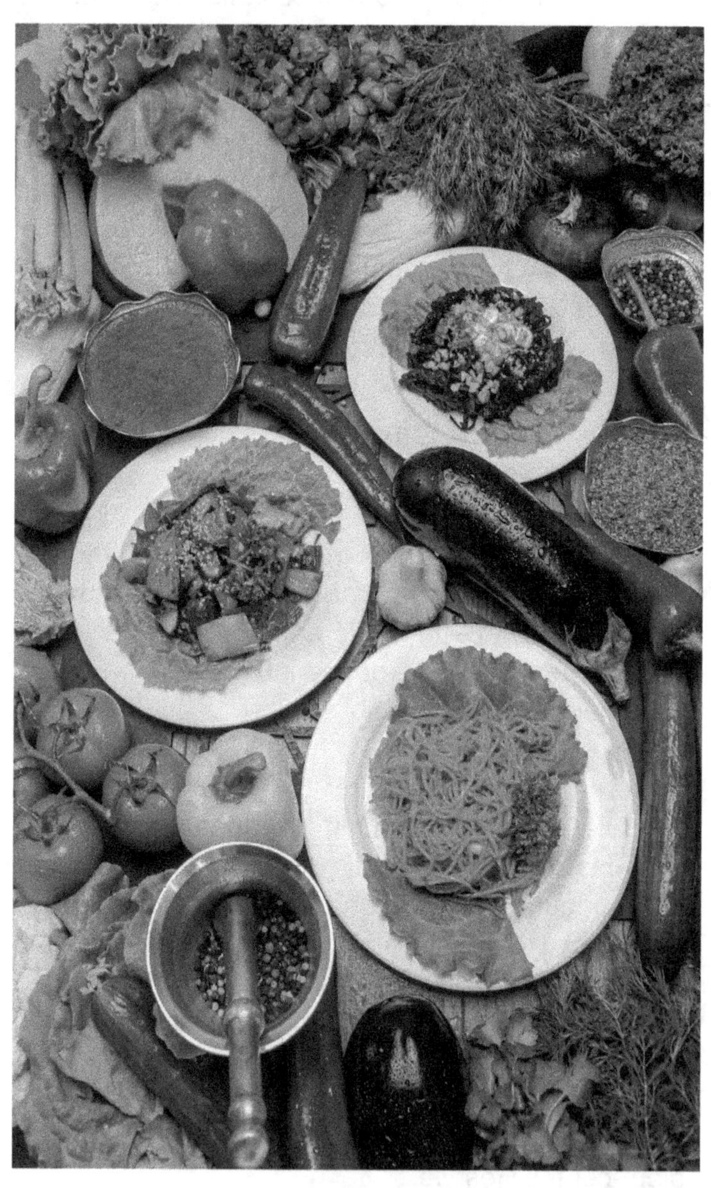

CHAPTER TWO

Nutritional Science Behind Plant-Based Diets.

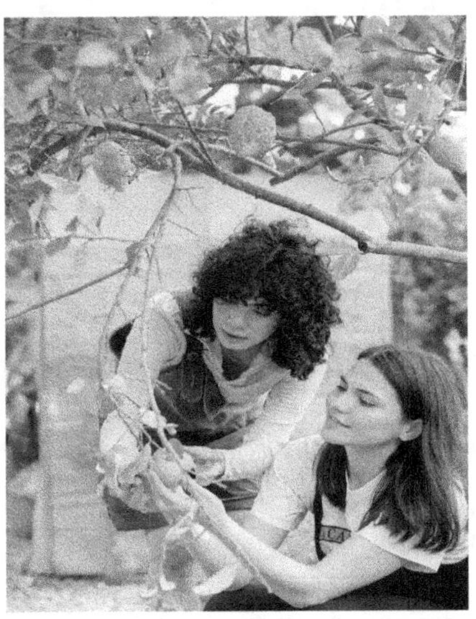

Embarking on the journey into the nutritional science behind plant-based diets unveils a captivating realm where the vibrancy of whole, plant-derived foods converges with the intricate tapestry of human health. Delving into this world reveals the potency of macronutrients, micronutrients, and phytochemicals within plant foods—illuminating the profound impact these elements wield in nourishing our bodies and fostering optimal well-being.

Macronutrients in Plant-Based Foods

Understanding the diverse range of macronutrients in plant-based foods and their sources underscores the importance of a well-rounded plant-based diet in meeting nutritional needs while promoting overall health and vitality.

We shall consider closely macronutrients in plant-based foods accordingly:

1. Carbohydrates:

Sources: Plant-based diets are abundant in carbohydrates derived from various sources such as fruits, vegetables, legumes, whole grains, and starchy vegetables like potatoes.

Types and Benefits:
Carbohydrates in plant foods encompass simple sugars (fructose, glucose) found in fruits, complex carbohydrates (fiber, starch) present in vegetables, grains, and legumes. These carbohydrates provide energy, aid in digestion, and offer a steady source of fuel for the body.

2. Proteins
Sources: Plant-based proteins are plentiful in legumes (beans, lentils, chickpeas), nuts, seeds, tofu, tempeh, whole grains, and certain vegetables like spinach and broccoli

Types and Benefits:
Plant proteins comprise essential and non-essential amino acids, vital for various bodily functions, including muscle repair and synthesis, enzyme production, and immune function. While some plant sources may lack specific amino acids, a varied plant-based diet ensures adequate protein intake and a balance of essential amino acids.

3. Fats

Sources:
Plant-based fats are found in avocados, nuts, seeds, olives, coconuts, and plant-based oils like olive oil, flaxseed oil, and avocado oil.

Types and Benefits:
Plant-based fats include monounsaturated and polyunsaturated fats, along with omega-3 and omega-6 fatty acids. These fats support heart health, brain function, hormone production, and absorption of fat-soluble vitamins. Incorporating a variety of plant-based fats ensures a balanced intake of healthy fats essential for overall well-being.

4. Fiber

Sources:
Fiber is abundant in plant-based foods such as fruits, vegetables, whole grains, legumes, nuts, and seeds.

Types and Benefits:
Plant-based diets are rich in dietary fiber, comprising soluble and insoluble fiber. Fiber aids in digestion, promotes satiety, regulates blood sugar levels, and supports a healthy gut microbiome. It also contributes to reducing the risk of chronic diseases, including heart disease, diabetes, and certain cancers.

5. Micronutrients

Sources:
Plant-based foods are dense with essential micronutrients like vitamins (A, C, K, E, B-complex vitamins) and minerals (iron, calcium, magnesium, potassium) found in various fruits, vegetables, nuts, seeds, and whole grains.

Types and Benefits:
These micronutrients play pivotal roles in various bodily functions, from supporting immune health, bone strength, and energy metabolism to acting as antioxidants, aiding in cell repair, and combating oxidative stress.

Micronutrients and Phytochemicals

Micronutrients:

Micronutrients are essential nutrients that the body requires in smaller quantities compared to macronutrients (carbohydrates, proteins, and fats) but are equally vital for various physiological functions, growth, and overall health.

Types of Micronutrients:

1. Vitamins:

These are organic compounds that are crucial for various bodily functions and are typically obtained from diet or supplements. They are classified into water-soluble vitamins (e.g., Vitamin C and B-complex vitamins) and fat-soluble vitamins (e.g., Vitamins A, D, E, and K).

2. Minerals:

Minerals are inorganic compounds necessary for bodily functions such as bone health, enzyme activity, and fluid balance. They include macrominerals (e.g., calcium, magnesium, potassium) required in larger amounts and trace minerals (e.g., iron, zinc, selenium) needed in smaller quantities.

Functions of Micronutrients:

- **Support Metabolism:**

Micronutrients participate in metabolic processes, helping enzymes catalyze reactions involved in energy production, cellular repair, and growth.

- **Enhance Immunity:**

Certain vitamins and minerals contribute to immune function, aiding in the body's defense against infections and diseases.

- **Bone Health and Tissue Maintenance:**

Micronutrients like calcium, Vitamin D, and magnesium are essential for bone strength and tissue repair.

- **Antioxidant Activities:**

Some micronutrients, such as Vitamin C, Vitamin E, and selenium, act as antioxidants, helping neutralize harmful free radicals and reducing oxidative stress in the body.

Phytochemicals:

Phytochemicals are naturally occurring compounds found in plant-based foods that have various health-promoting properties. They are not considered essential nutrients but have demonstrated significant benefits for human health.

Types and Sources:

★ Polyphenols:
Found in fruits, vegetables, tea, and red wine,
polyphenols exhibit antioxidant and
anti-inflammatory properties.

★ Carotenoids:
These are pigments responsible for the vibrant
colors in fruits and vegetables. Examples include
beta-carotene in carrots and lycopene in tomatoes,
known for their antioxidant effects.

★ Flavonoids:
Present in various fruits, vegetables, and herbs,
flavonoids have anti-inflammatory, anti-cancer, and
antioxidant properties

Health Benefits:

● Antioxidant Effects:
Phytochemicals often act as antioxidants,
protecting cells from damage caused by free
radicals, thus reducing the risk of chronic diseases.

● Anti-inflammatory Properties:
Some phytochemicals exhibit anti-inflammatory
effects, potentially reducing the risk of inflammatory
conditions like heart disease and arthritis.

- **Cancer Prevention:**

Certain phytochemicals have shown promise in inhibiting the growth of cancer cells and reducing the risk of certain cancers.

Incorporating a diverse range of plant-based foods rich in micronutrients and phytochemicals into the diet supports overall health and reduces the risk of chronic diseases.

Impact of Plant-Based Diets on Health

1. Cardiovascular Health:

Lower Risk of Heart Disease: Plant-based diets, rich in fruits, vegetables, whole grains, nuts, and seeds, have been associated with reduced risks of cardiovascular diseases due to their high fiber, antioxidants, and phytochemical content. They help lower blood pressure, cholesterol levels, and reduce the risk of strokes and heart attacks.

2. Weight Management:

Promotion of Healthy Weight: Plant-based diets are often lower in calories and saturated fats compared to animal-based diets, making them beneficial for weight management. Higher fiber content in plant-based foods also aids in feeling full, reducing overall calorie intake.

3. **Type 2 Diabetes Prevention and Management:**

Improved Insulin Sensitivity:Plant-based diets, particularly those rich in whole grains, legumes, fruits, and vegetables, have shown to improve insulin sensitivity, aiding in the prevention and management of type 2 diabetes.

4. **Cancer Prevention:**

Reduced Risk of Certain Cancers: High consumption of fruits, vegetables, and legumes is associated with a lower risk of certain cancers, attributed to the presence of antioxidants, phytochemicals, and fiber that help neutralize free radicals and reduce inflammation.

5. **Digestive Health:**

Improved Gut Health: Plant-based diets, especially those high in fiber-rich foods, support a healthy gut microbiome, promoting regular bowel movements and reducing the risk of gastrointestinal diseases like diverticulitis and colon cancer.

6. **Bone Health:**

Adequate Nutrient Intake: Although plant-based diets may lack certain bone-building nutrients like calcium and Vitamin D found in dairy and fish, they can provide adequate levels of these nutrients through fortified foods and supplements, contributing to bone health.

7. **Longevity and Overall Well-being:**
Reduced Inflammation: Plant-based diets have been associated with reduced systemic inflammation, which is linked to various chronic diseases. This anti-inflammatory effect contributes to overall health and longevity.

8. **Enhanced Vitality:**
The high nutrient content, antioxidants, and phytochemicals in plant-based foods can boost energy levels, improve mood, and enhance overall vitality.

9. **Environmental and Ethical Impact:**
Plant-based diets have a lower environmental footprint compared to animal-based diets, requiring fewer resources like water and land, and producing fewer greenhouse gas emissions.

Conclusion:
Plant-based diets, when well-planned and nutritionally balanced, have been extensively associated with numerous health benefits, including reduced risks of chronic diseases, weight management, improved gut health, and overall well-being. However, it's crucial to ensure adequate intake of essential nutrients like Vitamin B12, iron, calcium, and Omega-3 fatty acids commonly found in animal-based foods. A varied and balanced plant-based diet can significantly contribute to overall health while also benefiting the environment.

CHAPTER THREE

Transitioning to a Plant-Based Lifestyle

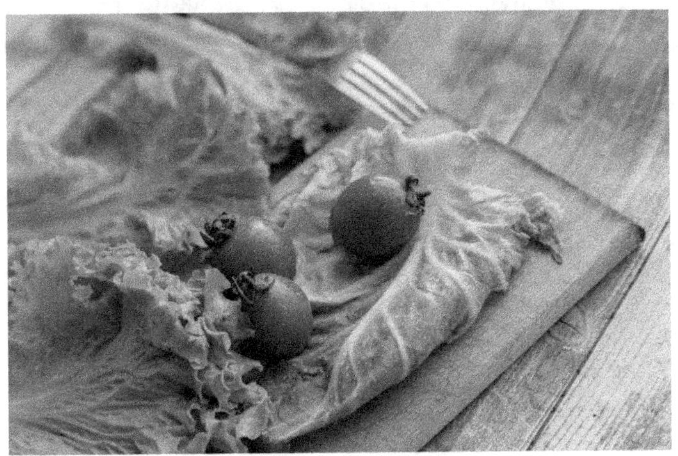

Overcoming Challenges

Transitioning to a plant-based lifestyle can be a rewarding and fulfilling journey, but it can also come with its fair share of challenges. In this chapter, you will explore some of the common obstacles people face when transitioning to a plant-based lifestyle and provide strategies to overcome them.

1. Lack of Knowledge:

One of the main challenges is the lack of knowledge and familiarity with plant-based foods. Many people may not know how to source, cook, or combine plant-based ingredients to create balanced and satisfying meals. To overcome this challenge, it is essential to educate yourself about plant-based nutrition and explore various plant-based recipes and meal ideas. There are numerous online resources, cookbooks, and communities that can provide guidance and support in this journey. Experimenting with different plant-based foods and flavors can also help expand your palate and make the transition more enjoyable. This knowledge helps in planning balanced meals and ensures you're meeting your dietary requirements.

2. Nutritional Deficiencies:

Ensuring adequate nutrition when transitioning to a plant-based lifestyle is vital. Some nutrients, such as vitamin B12, iron, calcium, and omega-3 fatty acids, may be less abundant in plant-based diets. It is crucial to be mindful of these nutrients and consume a wide variety of plant-based foods that provide them. Educate yourself about plant-based sources of key nutrients, and consider incorporating fortified foods or supplements as needed. Consulting with a registered dietitian or nutritionist who specializes in plant-based diets can provide personalized guidance to help meet your nutritional needs during the transition.

3. Social Pressures and Judgment:

Another common challenge is dealing with social pressures and potential judgment from family, friends, and acquaintances. Many individuals transitioning to a plant-based lifestyle may face criticism or encounter situations where their dietary choices are not accommodated in social gatherings. It's important to remember that everyone's dietary choices are personal, and it's crucial to stand firm in your decision. Seek support from like-minded individuals or join local plant-based communities or online forums to connect with people who understand and share your journey. Communicating your dietary needs with others in a respectful and informative manner can also help manage social situations and garner support.

4. Gradual Transition:

Instead of an abrupt shift, gradually incorporate more plant-based foods into your diet. Start by dedicating specific days or meals each week to plant-based options. Slowly reducing animal products allows your palate and body to adapt.

1. **Recipe Exploration and Variety:**
Explore diverse plant-based recipes to keep meals interesting and enjoyable. Experiment with different cuisines, ingredients, and cooking techniques. This variety prevents monotony and increases the chances of sticking to the new lifestyle.

2. **Meal Planning and Preparation:**
Plan meals in advance to ensure you have the necessary ingredients on hand. Batch cooking can be helpful, preparing larger quantities to freeze or use throughout the week. This minimizes the stress of meal preparation on busy days.

3. **Social Support and Resources:**
Seek support from like-minded individuals, whether through online communities, local meet-ups, or friends and family. Share experiences, recipes, and tips for a smoother transition. Additionally, utilize

cookbooks, websites, and documentaries focused on plant-based living for inspiration.

4. **Addressing Nutritional Gaps:**
Be mindful of essential nutrients like vitamin B12, iron, calcium, and omega-3 fatty acids, which may require supplementation or careful planning in a plant-based diet. Consulting a registered dietitian or healthcare professional can provide personalized guidance.

5. **Handling Social Situations:**
Eating out or attending social gatherings might pose challenges initially. However, most restaurants now offer plant-based options. When invited, communicate your dietary preferences politely and offer to bring a dish to share, ensuring there's something you can eat.

6. **Mindset Shift and Patience:**
Embrace a positive mindset and be patient with yourself during this transition. It's normal to face setbacks or cravings for familiar foods. Acknowledge your progress, focus on the benefits, and understand that it's a journey with room for adjustments.

7. **Environmental and Ethical Motivation:**
Remind yourself of the reasons behind your decision to adopt a plant-based lifestyle,

whether it's for environmental sustainability, animal welfare, or health. This motivation can reinforce your commitment during challenging times.

8. **Continuous Learning and Adaptation:** Stay open to learning new information and adapting your approach. As you progress, your tastes, cooking skills, and nutritional knowledge will evolve, allowing for a more sustainable and enjoyable plant-based lifestyle.

By addressing these challenges methodically and persistently, the transition to a plant-based lifestyle can become a fulfilling and sustainable choice.

Tips for Transitioning Gradually to plant-based diets.

Transitioning gradually to a plant-based diet is a practical and sustainable approach. Here's a detailed analysis of tips to facilitate this process:

1. Start with Meatless Days:
Designate specific days of the week as meatless. This allows you to experiment with plant-based meals without the pressure of an immediate full transition.

2. Explore Plant-Based Proteins:

Familiarize yourself with plant-based protein sources like legumes, beans, lentils, tofu, and tempeh. Experiment with these in your favorite recipes to find what you enjoy.

3. Emphasize Whole Foods:

Focus on whole, minimally processed foods. Incorporate a variety of fruits, vegetables, whole grains, nuts, and seeds into your meals for a well-rounded and nutrient-dense diet.

4. Educate Yourself:

Learn about the nutritional aspects of a plant-based diet. Understanding the importance of balancing macronutrients, getting essential vitamins and minerals, and meeting protein needs will help you make informed food choices.

5. Meal Swap Approach:

Gradually replace animal products in your meals with plant-based alternatives. For instance, try plant-based milk instead of dairy, or swap meat with beans in your favorite dishes. Over time, increase the proportion of plant-based components.

6. Experiment with Plant-Based Recipes:

Explore new recipes that showcase the diversity and flavors of plant-based ingredients. This not only adds excitement to your meals but also helps you discover enjoyable alternatives to traditional dishes.

7. **Build a Plant-Based Pantry:**

Stock up on plant-based staples such as grains, legumes, canned tomatoes, spices, and herbs. Having these items readily available simplifies meal preparation and encourages you to cook more plant-based meals at home.

8. **Learn Label Reading:**

Develop the habit of reading food labels to identify animal-derived ingredients. Understanding how to spot hidden animal products will empower you to make conscious choices while grocery shopping.

9. **Gradual Reduction of Animal Products:**

Gradually reduce the quantity of animal products in your meals. For instance, if you're used to having meat with every meal, start by having smaller portions or incorporating more plant-based sides.

10. **Listen to Your Body:**

Pay attention to how your body responds to the changes. If you experience cravings or feel fatigued, consider adjusting your diet to better meet your nutritional needs. Consult a healthcare professional or nutritionist for guidance if necessary.

11. **Connect with the Plant-Based Community:**

Join online forums, social media groups, or local communities that focus on plant-based living. Engaging with others who are on a similar journey can provide support, motivation, and valuable tips.

12. **Celebrate Successes:**
Acknowledge and celebrate your progress, no matter how small. Whether it's successfully trying a new plant-based recipe or going a full day without animal products, recognizing achievements reinforces positive behavior.

By adopting these tips and embracing a gradual mindset, you can smoothly transition to a plant-based diet while discovering enjoyable and sustainable eating habits.

Plant-based Meal Planning and Preparation

This session provides insights into the nuances of meal planning and preparation within the context of a plant-based diet, addressing nutritional needs, building balanced plates, and offering practical tips for successful adoption of this wholesome lifestyle.

Adopting a plant-based diet doesn't just involve a change in ingredients; it's a shift in lifestyle and a commitment to nourishing your body with the goodness of plant-derived foods. Successful adherence to a plant-based diet often hinges on thoughtful meal planning and strategic preparation. Let's explore the key aspects of meal planning and preparation tailored to the plant-based lifestyle.

1. **Understanding Nutritional Needs:**

a. **Essential Nutrients:**
  - Identify key nutrients in plant-based foods, including protein sources like beans and lentils, iron-rich greens, calcium in fortified plant milks, and Omega-3 fatty acids from flaxseeds and walnuts.

b. **Balancing Macronutrients:**
  - Plan meals with a balance of carbohydrates, proteins, and healthy fats. Incorporate a variety of whole grains, legumes, and nuts to ensure a diverse nutrient profile.

2. **Building a Balanced Plate:**
a. *Colorful Variety:*
  - Different colors in fruits and vegetables signify distinct antioxidants and phytochemicals, contributing to overall health.

b. *Plant-Based Protein:*
  - Include protein sources such as tofu, tempeh, legumes, and quinoa. Combining complementary protein sources enhances amino acid profiles.

c. *Healthy Fats:*
- Incorporate sources of healthy fats like avocados, nuts, and seeds for satiety and essential fatty acids.

3. **Weekly Meal Planning:**

a. *Batch Cooking:*
- Streamline your week by preparing batch staples like whole grains, roasted vegetables, and legumes. These versatile ingredients can be repurposed into various meals.

b. *Variety Across Days:*
- Ensure diversity throughout the week. Plan meals with different grains, proteins, and vegetables to avoid monotony and ensure a broad nutrient intake.

4. **Smart Shopping:**

a. *Seasonal and Local Produce:*
- Prioritize seasonal and locally sourced produce for freshness, flavor, and sustainability.

b. *Whole Foods Focus:*
- Shop the perimeter of the grocery store, focusing on whole foods and minimizing processed items.

5. **Meal Preparation Hacks:**

a. Pre-Cut and Wash:
- Spend time washing, chopping, and prepping vegetables and fruits in advance for quick and easy assembly during the week.

b. *Freezing Staples:*
- Freeze portions of cooked grains, beans, and soups for convenient, time-saving options on busy days.

6. **Mindful Eating:**

a. Intuitive Choices:
Practice mindful eating by paying rapt attention to your body's hunger and fullness cues. Choose whole, unprocessed foods to nourish your body.
b. Enjoying the Process:
Make mealtime an enjoyable ritual. Experiment with new recipes, savor flavors, and appreciate the journey toward a healthier lifestyle.

7. **Recipe Exploration:**

a. *Cookbook Inspiration:*
Explore plant-based cookbooks for creative recipes and meal ideas. Experiment with flavors and textures to keep your palate engaged.

b. **Online Resources:**

Utilize online platforms for inspiration. Many websites offer plant-based recipes catering to various tastes and dietary preferences.

Conclusion:
Embarking on a plant-based journey is a culinary adventure filled with nourishment, vitality, and sustainable choices. Thoughtful meal planning and preparation empower individuals to embrace the abundance of plant-derived goodness while making the transition to a plant-based lifestyle seamless and enjoyable.

Plant-Based Meal Planning and Preparation Schedule

Meal planning and preparation are essential for successfully adopting a plant-based lifestyle. Here's a detailed guide to help you create a comprehensive schedule:

Week 1: Preparation and Education.

Day 1-2:   Educate Yourself
- Research plant-based nutrition.
- Identify essential nutrients and their plant sources.
- Create a list of staple ingredients.

Day 3-4:   Kitchen Overhaul
- Clean out your pantry and refrigerator.
- Replace animal products with plant-based alternatives.
- Stock up on whole grains, legumes, nuts, seeds, and fresh produce.

Day 5-7:   Recipe Exploration
- Collect diverse plant-based recipes.
- Experiment with a simple plant-based breakfast and dinner.
- Note your favorite recipes for future use.

Week 2:   Basic Meal Structure

Day 8-10: Balanced Meal Planning
- Plan three balanced meals and two snacks each day.
- Incorporate a variety of colors and textures for nutrient diversity.
- Ensure meals contain protein, healthy fats, and complex carbohydrates.

Day 11-12: Grocery Shopping
- Create a well balanced shopping list based on your meal plan.
- Visit local markets or grocery stores to purchase fresh ingredients.
- Explore specialty stores for unique plant-based products.

Day 13-14: Batch Cooking

- Prepare large batches of staple items (grains, beans, sauces).
- Store in portions for easy use during the week.
- Freeze extra portions for a longer shelf life.

Week 3: Building Consistency

Day 15-17: Daily Routine Adjustment

- Establish a consistent mealtime routine.
- Incorporate plant-based snacks to maintain energy levels.
- Carefully observe how your body responds to this new eating schedule.

Day 18-19: Dining Out Strategies

- Research plant-based options at local restaurants.
- Learn to modify menu items to suit your preferences.
- Have a list of go-to restaurants that cater to plant-based diets.

Day 20-21: Recipe Refinement

- Fine-tune your favorite recipes based on taste preferences.
- Explore the use of herbs and spices for added flavor.
- Share successful recipes with friends or online communities.

Week 4: Sustainable Practices

Day 22 - 24: Sustainability Focus
- Explore local and seasonal produce options.
- Reduce food waste by repurposing leftovers.
- Incorporate reusable containers for meal storage.

Day 25 - 26: Nutrient Analysis
- Evaluate your nutrient intake through apps or nutrition guides.
- Adjust meal plans to address any nutritional gaps.
- You may also need to consult a nutritionist for personalized advice.

Day 27-28: Reflection and Adaptation
- Reflect on the past month's journey.
- Build on your successes and identify areas for improvement.
- Adjust your meal plan based on feedback and experience.

Ongoing: Continuous Improvement
- Monthly Review: Reassess and adjust your meal plan monthly.
- Seasonal Updates: Modify recipes based on seasonal produce availability.
-Recipe Expansion: Continuously explore new plant-based recipes.

By following this detailed plant-based meal planning and preparation schedule, you'll establish a foundation for a sustainable diet for yourself.

Part II: Health Benefits of Plant-Based Diets

CHAPTER FOUR

Heart Health and Plant-Based Eating

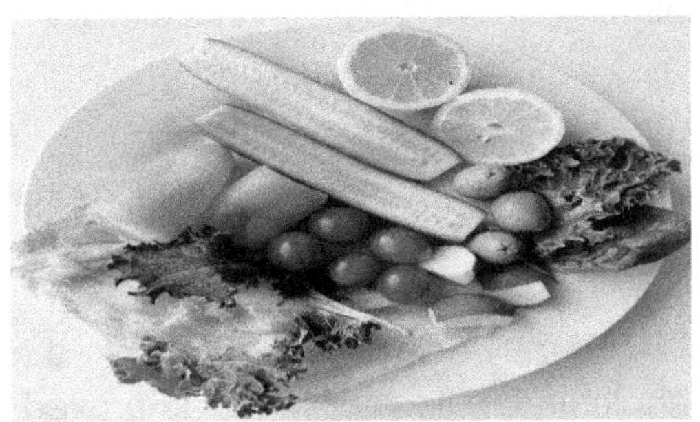

Lowering Cholesterol and Blood Pressure

Lowering cholesterol and blood pressure through a plant-based diet involves making strategic dietary choices. Here's a detailed analysis of how to achieve these goals:

Lowering Cholesterol:

1. Choose Heart-Healthy Fats:

- Prioritize sources of unsaturated fats, such as avocados, nuts, seeds, and olive oil.
- Reduce saturated fats by replacing animal fats with plant-based alternatives.

2. Increase Soluble Fiber Intake:

- Consume fiber-rich foods like oats, barley, beans, lentils, fruits, and vegetables.
- Soluble fiber helps lower LDL cholesterol by binding to it and aiding in its elimination.

3. Include Omega-3 Fatty Acids:

- Incorporate omega-3-rich foods like flaxseeds, chia seeds, walnuts, and algae-based supplements.
- These fatty acids have been linked to lower cholesterol levels and improved heart health.

4. Limit Processed Foods:

- Reduce intake of processed and refined foods, as they often contain trans fats and contribute to elevated cholesterol levels.

5. Increase Plant Sterols:

- Include foods fortified with plant sterols, like certain margarines and orange juice.

- Plant sterols can help block the absorption of cholesterol in the digestive system.

6. Eat More Plant-Based Proteins:

- Choose plant-based protein sources, such as tofu, tempeh, legumes, and quinoa.
- These proteins are generally lower in saturated fat compared to animal proteins.

7. Stay Hydrated:

- Drink plenty of water, as hydration supports overall cardiovascular health.
- Herbal teas, especially those with hibiscus, may have a positive impact on cholesterol levels.

Lowering Blood Pressure:

1. Increase Potassium Intake:

- Consume potassium-rich foods like bananas, oranges, sweet potatoes, and beans.

2. Limit Sodium Intake:

- Reduce processed and high-sodium foods, such as canned soups and salty snacks.
- Use spices and herbs for flavor in place of using excessive salt.

3. **Focus on Magnesium-Rich Foods:**
   - Include magnesium-rich foods like leafy greens, nuts, seeds, and whole grains.

   - Magnesium contributes to blood vessel relaxation, aiding in blood pressure regulation.

4. **Emphasize Plant-Based Diets (DASH):**
   - Follow the Dietary Approaches to Stop Hypertension (DASH) diet, which emphasizes fruits, vegetables, whole grains, and low-fat dairy.

5. **Maintain a Healthy Weight:**
   - Achieve and maintain a healthy weight through a plant-based diet and regular physical activity.

   - Weight loss can significantly impact blood pressure levels.

6. **Stay Active:**
   - Exercise contributes to lower blood pressure and overall cardiovascular health.

7. **Moderate Alcohol Consumption:**
   - Excessive alcohol intake can raise blood pressure; limit it to recommended levels.

8. **Manage Stress:**
- Chronic stress can contribute to elevated blood pressure.

Adopting a plant-based diet that incorporates these strategies can effectively lower cholesterol and blood pressure, promoting long-term heart health. It's crucial to consult with a healthcare professional for personalized advice and monitoring.

Preventing Cardiovascular Diseases

Preventing cardiovascular diseases through a plant-based diet involves adopting a lifestyle that prioritizes heart-healthy food choices. Here's a detailed analysis of how to leverage a plant-based diet for cardiovascular health:

Foundation of a Plant-Based Diet for Cardiovascular Health:

1. **Emphasize Whole Plant Foods:**

- Maintain regular intake of fruits, vegetables, whole grains, legumes, nuts, and seeds.

- These foods are rich in fiber, antioxidants, vitamins, and minerals crucial for heart health.

2. **Choose Healthy Fats:**
- Go for unsaturated fats in avocados, olive oil, and nuts.

- Limit saturated and trans fats commonly found in animal products and processed foods.

3. **Increase Fiber Intake:**
- Consume a variety of fiber-rich foods to support digestion and lower cholesterol.

- Whole grains, beans, lentils, fruits, and vegetables are excellent sources of dietary fiber.

4. **Include Omega-3 Fatty Acids:**
- Omega-3s contribute to cardiovascular health by reducing inflammation and improving lipid profiles.

5. **Limit Processed Foods and Added Sugars:**
- Minimize intake of processed foods, sugary beverages, and dessert.

- These can contribute to weight gain, inflammation, and increased risk of cardiovascular diseases.

Key Strategies for Cardiovascular Disease Prevention:

1. **Monitor Sodium Intake:**
   - Reduce reliance on high-sodium processed foods.
   - Use herbs, spices, and other flavorings to season meals instead of excessive salt.

2. **Follow the DASH Diet Principles:**
   - Adopt principles from the Dietary Approaches to Stop Hypertension (DASH) diet.
   - Take more fruits, vegetables, lean proteins, and low-fat dairy while reducing sodium intake

3. **Maintain a Healthy Weight:**
   - Strive for and maintain a healthy weight through a balanced plant-based diet and regular exercise.
   - Weight management is crucial for reducing the risk of cardiovascular diseases.

4. **Regular Physical Activity:**
   - Engage in at least 150 minutes of moderate-intensity aerobic exercise per week.
   - Exercise promotes heart health, helps manage weight, and lowers blood pressure.

5. **Moderate Alcohol Consumption:**

- Moderate alcohol intake, particularly red wine, relates to some cardiovascular benefits.

6. Manage Stress:
- Adopt stress-reducing practices such as meditation, yoga, or deep breathing exercises.
- Chronic stress can contribute to cardiovascular issues.

7. Regular Health Check-ups:
- Schedule regular health check-ups with a physician to be in control of health.
- Monitor blood pressure, cholesterol levels, and other cardiovascular risk factors.

8. Quit Smoking:
- Smoking is a major risk factor for cardiovascular diseases; quitting significantly improves heart health.

9. Stay Hydrated:
- Drink an adequate amount of water daily to support overall cardiovascular health.
- Proper hydration aids in blood circulation and helps maintain optimal heart function.

By adopting a plant-based diet and incorporating these lifestyle strategies, you can significantly reduce the risk of cardiovascular diseases.

CHAPTER FIVE

Managing Weight
with Plant-Based Diets

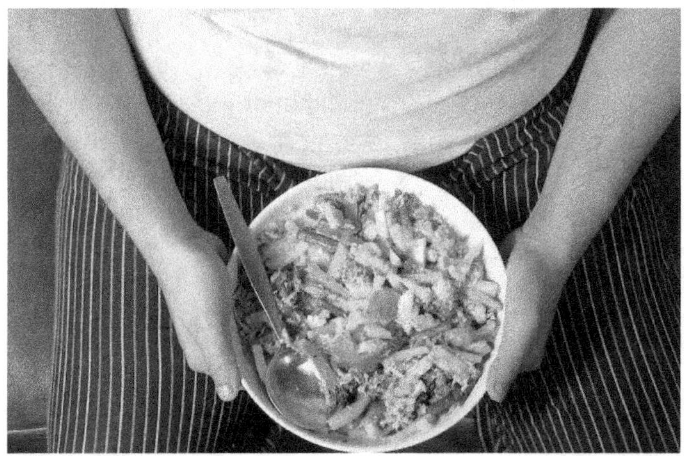

Weight Loss Strategies

*Strategies for Effective Weight Loss with
Plant-Based Diets.*

Achieving and maintaining a healthy weight through
a plant-based diet involves strategic planning and
mindful choices. In this chapter, Andrea Rich distills
effective strategies for weight loss with plant-based
diets:

1. Emphasize Whole, Plant-Based Foods:

a. Abundance of Fruits and Vegetables:
Make it a priority to take a variety of fruits and vegetables. They are rich in fiber, vitamins, and minerals while being low in calories, making them ideal for weight loss.

b. Whole Grains and Legumes:
Incorporate whole grains like quinoa, brown rice, and oats, along with legumes such as beans and lentils, they provide sustained energy and promote a feeling of satisfaction.

2. Mindful Portion Control:
a. Use Smaller Plates:
Opt for smaller plates to encourage controlled portion sizes. This strategy can help prevent overeating.

b. Listen to Hunger Cues:
Monitor your body's hunger from time to time and fullness signals. Eat slowly and savor each bite to allow your body time to register fullness.

3. Optimize Plant-Based Protein Sources:
a. Diverse Protein Choices:
Include a variety of plant-based protein sources such as tofu, tempeh, seitan, legumes, and edamame. Protein promotes satiety and supports muscle maintenance during weight loss.

b. Strategic Protein Timing:
- Distribute protein intake throughout the day to maintain muscle mass and enhance metabolism.

4. Choose Healthy Fats Wisely:

a. Focus on Monounsaturated and Polyunsaturated Fats:
leverage on sources of healthy fats like avocados, nuts, seeds, and olive oil. Cut down intake of saturated and trans fats found in processed foods.

b. Mindful Fat Portions:
Be mindful of portion sizes for calorie-dense fats. While healthy, they contribute to overall caloric intake.

5. Limit Processed Foods:
a. Minimize Refined Carbohydrates:
Limit your consumption rate of refined carbohydrates and processed foods. Opt for whole, minimally processed options for sustained energy.

b. Watch Added Sugars:
Be aware of added sugars in plant-based products. Choose whole fruits over sugary snacks.

6. Hydrate Effectively:
a. Water as a Primary Beverage:
Adopt the use of water as the main beverage throughout the day. It aids digestion and can help prevent overeating.

b. Herbal Teas and Infusions:
Include herbal teas and infusions as calorie-free alternatives to sugary or high-calorie beverages.

7. Regular Physical Activity:

a. Incorporate Cardiovascular Exercise:
Include aerobic exercises like brisk walking, cycling, or swimming to burn calories and support overall health.

b. Strength Training for Muscle Maintenance:
Incorporate strength training exercises to maintain and build lean muscle mass, contributing to a higher metabolism.

8. Plan Balanced Meals:

a. Varied and Colorful Plates:
Aim for colorful, varied meals with a mix of vegetables, fruits, whole grains, and plant-based proteins.

b. Strategic Meal Timing:
Plan meals and snacks to avoid prolonged periods without food. It helps to regulate blood sugar levels and prevent excessive hunger.

9. Keep a Food Journal:
a. Record Daily Intake:
Maintain a food journal to track meals and snacks. This can enhance awareness of eating patterns and identify areas for improvement.
b. Monitor Emotional Eating:
Identify and address emotional eating by noting triggers and finding alternative coping mechanisms.

10. Seek Professional Guidance:

a. Consult a Registered Dietitian:
If needed, seek guidance from a registered dietitian or nutritionist experienced in plant-based diets. Personalized advice can optimize weight loss efforts.

Conclusion:

Effective weight loss with a plant-based diet involves a holistic approach, combining nutrient-dense food choices, mindful eating practices, regular physical activity, and strategic planning. By adopting these strategies, individuals can harness the benefits of a plant-based lifestyle for sustainable and healthy weight management.

Sustaining Healthy Weight

Strategies for Sustaining a Healthy Weight with a Plant-Based Diet

Maintaining a healthy weight is not only about losing pounds but sustaining a lifestyle that supports overall well-being. Here's are some strategies for sustaining a healthy weight with a plant-based diet:

1. Nutrient-Rich Plant Foods:

a. Diverse Fruits and Vegetables:

- Ensure a colorful array of fruits and vegetables to obtain a wide range of essential nutrients. This supports overall health and provides natural sweetness to curb cravings for processed sweets.

b. Whole Grains and Legumes:

- Embrace whole grains like quinoa, brown rice, and whole wheat, combined with legumes such as lentils and chickpeas for sustained energy and satiety.

2. Balanced Macronutrient Intake:

a. Plant-Based Proteins:

- Opt for diverse plant-based protein sources like tofu, tempeh, beans, and edamame to support muscle maintenance and overall metabolic health.

b. Healthy Fats:

- Include sources of healthy fats such as avocados, nuts, seeds, and olive oil in moderation to provide essential nutrients and enhance satiety.

3. Mindful Eating Practices:

a. Conscious Mealtime:

- Practice mindful eating by savoring each bite, appreciating flavors, and avoiding distractions. This fosters a better connection with hunger and fullness cues.

b. Intuitive Choices:

- Listen to your body's signals. Eat when hungry and stop when satisfied. This promotes a sustainable and natural approach to managing food intake.

4. Consistent Physical Activity:

a. Enjoyable Exercise Routine:

- Engage in physical activities you enjoy, whether it's dancing, hiking, or yoga. Consistency is key for sustained weight management.

b. Mix Cardio and Strength Training:

- Combine cardiovascular exercises with strength training to maintain muscle mass, boost metabolism, and support overall fitness.

5. Hydration as a Habit:

a. Regular Water Intake:

- Adopt the use of water as your primary beverage all day long. Staying well-hydrated supports metabolism and can sometimes be mistaken for hunger.

b. Infused Water and Herbal Teas:

- Add variety with infused water or herbal teas to make hydration enjoyable without added calories.

6. Meal Planning and Preparation:

a. Balanced Meal Structure:

- Plan well-balanced meals with a mix of vegetables, plant proteins, whole grains, and healthy fats. This avoids last-minute unhealthy choices.

b. Batch Cooking for Convenience:

- Embrace batch cooking to have wholesome, plant-based meals readily available, reducing the temptation of less healthy options.

7. Regular Health Check-ins:

a. Regular Health Assessments:

- Schedule regular check-ups to monitor health indicators such as blood pressure, cholesterol, and body composition. This provides insights into overall well-being.

b. Adjustments as Needed:

- Be open to adjusting dietary and lifestyle habits based on health assessments. Personalizing your approach ensures sustainability.

8. Culinary Exploration:

a. Varied and Exciting Meals:

- Keep your plant-based diet exciting by exploring new recipes and cuisines. This prevents monotony and makes the lifestyle enjoyable.

b. Seasonal and Local Ingredients:

- Embrace seasonal and local produce for freshness, variety, and to align with sustainable practices.

9. Emotional Well-being:

a. Stress Management Techniques:

- Adopt suitable stress management techniques that benefit your personality such as yoga, meditation, or deep breathing exercises. Emotional well-being is integral to sustaining a healthy lifestyle.

b. Mindful Indulgences:

- Allow occasional indulgences without guilt. Enjoying treats in moderation contributes to a balanced and sustainable approach to eating.

10. Community Support:

a. Join Plant-Based Communities

- Connect with like-minded individuals in plant-based communities. Sharing experiences, recipes, and tips provides support and motivation.

b. Educational Resources:

- Stay informed through reputable educational resources on plant-based nutrition. Continuous learning fosters a deeper understanding and commitment.

Conclusion:

Sustaining a healthy weight with a plant-based diet involves a multifaceted approach that extends beyond food choices. By incorporating nutrient-rich plant foods, embracing mindful eating, maintaining physical activity, and addressing emotional well-being, individuals can foster a lifestyle that promotes sustained health and vitality.

CHAPTER SIX

Enhancing Gut Health and Digestion

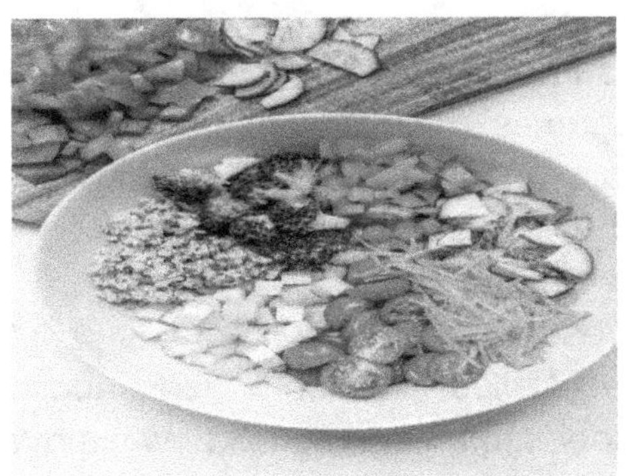

FIBER AND GUT MICROBIOME

A thriving gut is the cornerstone of overall well-being, and the dynamic interplay between dietary fiber and the gut microbiome plays a pivotal role. Here's a guide on how to enhance gut health and digestion through a synergistic approach involving fiber and the gut microbiome:

1. Understanding the Gut Microbiome:

a. Microbial Diversity:

- A diverse gut microbiome, consisting of trillions of bacteria, fungi, and viruses, is essential for optimal gut function and overall health.

b. *Microbial Balance:*
- Maintaining a balance between beneficial and potentially harmful microbes is crucial for digestive health and immune function.

2. The Role of Fiber:

a. Types of Dietary Fiber:

Soluble Fiber:
- Found in fruits, vegetables, oats, and legumes, soluble fiber forms a gel-like substance, aiding in digestion and nutrient absorption.

Insoluble Fiber:
- Present in whole grains, nuts, and vegetables, insoluble fiber adds bulk to stool, promoting regular bowel movements.

b. Prebiotic Fiber:
- Prebiotics, a type of fiber, serve as fuel for beneficial gut bacteria, promoting their growth and activity. Sources include garlic, onions, bananas, and asparagus.

3. Impact of Fiber on Gut Microbiome:

a. Increased Microbial Diversity:
- Diets rich in diverse fibers support a wide array of gut bacteria, contributing to increased microbial diversity.

b. Short-Chain Fatty Acids (SCFAs):
- Fermentation of fiber by gut bacteria produces SCFAs, such as butyrate, propionate, and acetate, which nourish colon cells and support gut health.

4. Strategies to Enhance Gut Health:
a. Gradual Increase in Fiber Intake:
- Gradually introduce higher fiber foods to allow the gut microbiome to adjust, preventing potential digestive discomfort.

b. Hydration:
- Ensure adequate hydration when increasing fiber intake. Water helps fiber move through the digestive system, preventing constipation.

5. Sources of Gut-Enhancing Fiber:
a. Colorful Vegetables and Fruits:
- A variety of colorful vegetables and fruits provide an array of fibers and antioxidants that nourish the gut.

b. Whole Grains and Legumes:
- Incorporate whole grains like brown rice, quinoa, and legumes such as lentils and chickpeas for a fiber-rich diet.

6. Fermented Foods:

a. Probiotic-Rich Options:
- Include fermented foods like yogurt, kefir, sauerkraut, and kimchi to introduce beneficial probiotics that support gut health.

b. Combining Prebiotics and Probiotics:
- Pair prebiotic-rich foods with probiotic sources for a synergistic effect, promoting the growth of beneficial bacteria.

7. Lifestyle Factors:

a. Regular Physical Activity:
- Exercise has been linked to a more diverse gut microbiome. Incorporate regular physical activity for overall health, including gut health.

b. Adequate Sleep:
- Prioritize quality sleep as it influences the gut-brain axis, impacting gut health and digestion.

8. Minimizing Processed Foods:

a. Reducing Added Sugars:
- Processed foods high in added sugars can negatively impact the gut microbiome. Always ensure you go for whole, unprocessed foods whenever possible.

b. Limiting Artificial Additives:

- Artificial additives in processed foods may disrupt the balance of the gut microbiome. Choose natural, whole-food options.

9. Monitoring Gut Health:

a. Pay Attention to Digestive Symptoms:

- Be aware of digestive symptoms such as bloating, gas, or irregular bowel movements. These can be indicators of gut health.

b. Consider Professional Guidance:

- Consult with a healthcare professional or registered dietitian if experiencing persistent digestive issues or before making significant dietary changes.

10. Continuous Adaptation:

a. Personalized Approach:

- Recognize that optimal gut health varies among individuals. Experiment with different fibers and dietary patterns to find what works best for your body.

b. Adapt to Changing Needs:

- The gut microbiome adapts to changes in diet and lifestyle. Be open to adjusting your approach based on your evolving health needs.

Conclusion:

The synergy between dietary fiber and the gut microbiome is a dynamic relationship that profoundly influences gut health and digestion. By incorporating a variety of fiber-rich foods, embracing fermented options, and considering lifestyle factors, individuals can foster an environment that supports a flourishing gut microbiome and overall well-being.

Addressing Digestive Issues

Digestive issues can significantly impact overall well-being, but a strategic approach can help address these concerns and enhance gut health. Here's a detailed analysis of how to tackle digestive issues for improved gastrointestinal function:

1. Identify and Understand Symptoms:

a. Recording Symptoms:
- Keep a detailed record of digestive symptoms, including frequency, intensity, and any patterns associated with specific foods or activities.

b. Common Digestive Issues:
- Recognize common digestive problems such as bloating, gas, constipation, diarrhea, and abdominal discomfort.

2. Gradual Introduction of Fiber:

a. Slow Increase in Fiber:

- Gradually introduce higher-fiber foods to prevent overwhelming the digestive system. This allows the gut to adapt gradually.

b. Balanced Fiber Sources:

- Include a mix of soluble and insoluble fiber from fruits, vegetables, whole grains, and legumes for comprehensive gut health.

3. Hydration and Fluid Intake:

a. Adequate Water Consumption:

- Ensure sufficient hydration, as water aids in the smooth passage of fiber through the digestive tract.

b. Limit Caffeine and Alcohol:

- Moderate caffeine and alcohol intake, as excessive consumption can contribute to dehydration and exacerbate digestive issues.

4. Introduce Fermented Foods:

a. Probiotic-Rich Options

- Include fermented foods like yogurt, kefir, sauerkraut, and kimchi to introduce beneficial probiotics that support a healthy gut microbiome.

b. Monitoring Reactions:

- Observe how the digestive system responds to fermented foods. Some individuals may need to introduce these gradually.

5. Probiotic Supplements:

a. Consultation with Healthcare Professional:

- Consider probiotic supplements under the guidance of a healthcare professional, especially if experiencing chronic digestive issues.

b. Strain-Specific Probiotics:

- Choose probiotic supplements with strains known to address specific digestive concerns, such as Lactobacillus and Bifidobacterium species.

6. Elimination Diet:

a. Identifying Trigger Foods:

- Consider an elimination diet to identify potential trigger foods that may exacerbate digestive issues. Reintroduce eliminated foods one at a time to observe reactions.

b. Professional Guidance:

- Seek guidance from a registered dietitian or healthcare professional when undertaking an elimination diet to ensure nutritional adequacy.

7. Mindful Eating Practices:

a. Chewing Thoroughly:

- Practice mindful eating by chewing food thoroughly. This helps a lot in the initial breakdown of food and supports digestion.

b. Avoiding Overeating:

- Consume meals in moderate portions to prevent overloading the digestive system.

8. Stress Management:

a. Mind-Body Techniques:

- Incorporate stress management techniques such as deep breathing, meditation, or yoga, as stress can exacerbate digestive issues.

b. Regular Physical Activity:

- Engage in regular physical activity, which can contribute to stress reduction and promote digestive health.

9. Identify Food Sensitivities:

a. Food Sensitivity Testing:

- Consider food sensitivity testing to identify potential triggers contributing to digestive discomfort.

b. Journaling and Observation:
- Keep a food journal to track reactions to specific foods and identify patterns over time.

10. Medical Evaluation:

a. Consulting Healthcare Professionals:
- If digestive issues persist, consult healthcare professionals such as gastroenterologists for a comprehensive evaluation and diagnosis.

b. Tests and Imaging:
- Diagnostic tests, including blood work, endoscopy, or imaging studies, may be recommended to identify underlying digestive conditions.

Conclusion:

Addressing digestive issues requires a personalized and comprehensive approach. By gradually introducing fiber, incorporating fermented foods, practicing mindful eating, managing stress, and seeking professional guidance when needed, individuals can enhance gut health and promote optimal digestion.

CHAPTER SEVEN

Diabetes Management and Plant-Based Diets

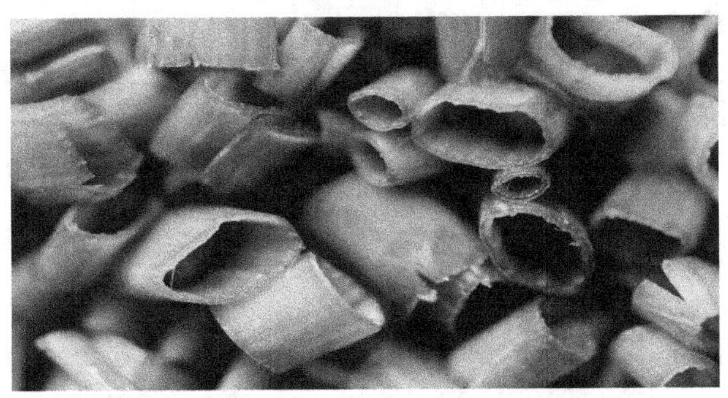

Controlling Blood Sugar Levels

Managing blood sugar levels is crucial for individuals with diabetes, and adopting a plant-based diet can be a powerful tool. Here are some proven strategies to control blood sugar levels effectively:

1. Emphasize Whole, Plant-Based Foods:
a. High-Fiber Choices:
- Prioritize fiber-rich foods like fruits, vegetables, whole grains, legumes, and nuts. Fiber slows glucose absorption, stabilizing blood sugar levels.

b. Low-Glycemic Index Foods:

- Opt for foods with a low glycemic index (GI), as they cause a slower rise in blood sugar. Examples include oats, quinoa, and most non-starchy vegetables.

2. Balanced Meal Planning:

a. Carbohydrate Distribution:

- Spread carbohydrate intake evenly throughout the day to prevent large spikes in blood sugar levels.

b. Protein Inclusion:

- Include plant-based protein sources like tofu, tempeh, beans, and legumes to promote satiety and stabilize blood sugar.

3. Portion Control and Monitoring:

a. Mindful Portion Sizes:

- Practice portion control to manage caloric intake and prevent excessive carbohydrate consumption.

b. Regular Blood Sugar Monitoring:

- Monitor blood sugar levels regularly to understand how different foods and meals affect glucose levels.

4. Choose Healthy Fats Wisely:

a. Heart-Healthy Fats:

- Incorporate sources of healthy fats like avocados, nuts, seeds, and olive oil in moderation. These fats support overall health.

b. Limit Saturated and Trans Fats:

- Minimize saturated and trans fats found in processed and fried foods, as they may contribute to insulin resistance.

5. Opt for Whole, Unprocessed Foods:

a. Minimize Processed Foods:

- Reduce intake of processed foods, which often contain hidden sugars and unhealthy additives.

b.Read Labels Carefully:

- Check food labels for hidden sugars, artificial sweeteners, and refined carbohydrates.

6. Hydration and Beverage Choices:

a. Water as Primary Beverage:

- Adopt the use of water as the main beverage to stay hydrated without added sugars.

b. Limit Sugary Drinks:

- Avoid sugary drinks and fruit juices, as they can lead to rapid spikes in blood sugar levels.

7. Regular Physical Activity:

a. Aerobic Exercise:

- Engage in regular aerobic exercises like walking, cycling, or swimming to improve insulin sensitivity and help manage blood sugar levels.

b. Strength Training:

- Include strength training exercises to build muscle mass, which aids in glucose metabolism.

8. Include Blood Sugar-Stabilizing Herbs and Spices:

a. Cinnamon and Turmeric:

- Incorporate cinnamon and turmeric into meals, as they may have blood sugar-lowering properties.

b. Fenugreek Seeds:

- Fenugreek seeds, when included in the diet, may help lower blood sugar levels.

9. Consideration of Individual Carbohydrate Tolerance:

a. Personalized Approach:

- Understand individual carbohydrate tolerance and adjust intake accordingly. Some may benefit from lower-carb approaches.

b. Consult with a Dietitian:
- Seek guidance from a registered dietitian to create a personalized meal plan based on individual needs and preferences.

10. Stress Management:

a. Mindfulness and Relaxation Techniques:
- Practice mindfulness, meditation, or other stress-relieving techniques, as stress can impact blood sugar levels.

b. Adequate Sleep:
- Ensure sufficient and quality sleep, as sleep deprivation can affect insulin sensitivity.

Key Principles of a Plant-Based Diet for Diabetes Management:

1. Emphasize Whole, Unprocessed Foods:
- Prioritize fruits, vegetables, whole grains, legumes, nuts, and seeds.

- These foods provide essential nutrients and fiber, slowing down the absorption of sugar.

2. Choose Low-Glycemic Index Foods:
- Opt for foods with a low glycemic index to prevent rapid spikes in blood sugar levels Examples include non-starchy vegetables, legumes, and most whole grains.

3. Portion Control and Balanced Meals:

- Pay attention to portion sizes to avoid overeating.

- Aim for balanced meals with a mix of carbohydrates, proteins, and healthy fats.

4. Healthy Carbohydrate Choices:

- Choose complex carbohydrates like whole grains (quinoa, brown rice), legumes, and high-fiber vegetables.

- Drastically reduce intake of refined carbohydrates and processed sugars.

5. Favor Plant-Based Proteins:

- Include plant-based protein sources such as tofu, tempeh, beans, lentils, and edamame.

- Plant-based proteins have a lower impact on blood sugar levels compared to animal proteins.

6. Healthy Fats:

- Prioritize sources of healthy fats like avocados, nuts, seeds, and olive oil.

- Limit saturated and trans fats found in animal products and processed foods.

7. Regular Meal Timing:

- Establish a consistent meal schedule to regulate blood sugar levels.

- Avoid skipping meals, and consider smaller, more frequent meals if needed.

8. Limit Added Sugars:

- Read food labels to identify hidden sugars in processed products.

- Use natural sweeteners like stevia or small amounts of maple syrup when necessary.

9. Hydration:

- Stay well-hydrated with water throughout the day.

- Limit sugary beverages, including fruit juices, which can lead to rapid blood sugar spikes.

Additional Strategies for Diabetes Management:

10. Monitor Blood Sugar Levels:

- Regularly check blood sugar levels as advised by healthcare professionals.

- Monitoring helps you understand the impact of different foods on your blood sugar.

11. Exercise Regularly:

- Engage in regular physical activity, including aerobic exercises and strength training.

- Regular body exercise improves insulin sensitivity and helps control blood sugar levels.

12. Regular Health Check-ups:

- Do remember to schedule regular check-ups with healthcare professionals.

- Keep track of other health parameters such as blood pressure and cholesterol.

13. Collaborate with Healthcare Professionals:

- Work closely with healthcare providers, including registered dietitians and endocrinologists.

- Personalized advice and regular follow-ups are crucial for effective diabetes management.

15. Gradual Transition:

- If transitioning to a plant-based diet is new, make gradual changes.

- This approach allows for adaptation and ensures long-term sustainability.

Conclusion:

Controlling blood sugar levels with a plant-based diet involves a holistic approach, combining nutrient-dense foods, mindful eating, regular physical activity, and individualized strategies. By adopting these comprehensive measures, individuals with diabetes can effectively manage blood sugar levels and support overall health.

Benefits of Plant-Based Diets for Type 2 Diabetes

Adopting a plant-based diet offers numerous advantages for individuals with Type 2 Diabetes, providing a holistic approach to managing the condition. Here are some of the benefits:

1. Improved Blood Sugar Control:
a. Fiber-Rich Foods:
- Plant-based diets, abundant in fruits, vegetables, whole grains, and legumes, are naturally high in fiber. Fiber slows the absorption of glucose, promoting stable blood sugar levels.

b. Low-Glycemic Index Foods:
- Emphasizing low-glycemic index foods helps prevent rapid spikes in blood sugar, supporting better glycemic control.

2. Enhanced Insulin Sensitivity:

a. Plant-Based Proteins:
- Protein sources from plants, such as beans, lentils, and tofu, contribute to improved insulin sensitivity, aiding glucose utilization.

b. Healthy Fats:
- Inclusion of heart-healthy fats from sources like avocados and nuts supports insulin function and metabolic health.

3. Weight Management:

a. Whole, Nutrient-Dense Foods:
- Plant-based diets are often lower in calories while being rich in essential nutrients.

- This promotes weight loss or maintenance, a key factor in managing Type 2 Diabetes.

b. Increased Satiety:
- High-fiber content and balanced macronutrients in plant-based meals contribute to increased feelings of fullness, assisting in portion control and weight management.

4. Cardiovascular Health:

a. Cholesterol Reduction:

- Plant-based diets have been linked to lower levels of LDL cholesterol, reducing the risk of   cardiovascular complications associated with Type 2 Diabetes.

b. Blood Pressure Control:

- The emphasis on potassium-rich foods in plant-based diets supports blood pressure regulation, crucial for individuals with diabetes.

5. Inflammation Reduction:

a. Anti-Inflammatory Properties:

- Plant-based foods, especially those rich in antioxidants and phytochemicals, contribute to an anti-inflammatory environment, potentially reducing inflammation associated with diabetes.

b. Omega-3 Fatty Acids:

- Inclusion of plant-based sources of omega-3 fatty acids, like flaxseeds and walnuts, may have anti-inflammatory effects.

6. Gut Microbiome Health:

a. Fiber for Gut Health:
  - The high fiber content of plant-based diets promotes a healthy gut microbiome, potentially influencing glucose metabolism and overall health.
b. Prebiotic Rich Foods:
  - Prebiotic foods like garlic, onions, and bananas nourish beneficial gut bacteria, contributing to a balanced gut ecosystem.

7. Reduced Risk of Complications:

a. Prevention of Diabetes-Related Complications:
- Managing blood sugar levels and promoting overall health through a plant-based diet may reduce the risk of complications such as neuropathy, nephropathy, and retinopathy.

b. *Lower Risk of Cardiovascular Events:*
- The cardiovascular benefits associated with plant-based diets contribute to a lower risk of heart-related complications.

8. Sustainable Lifestyle:

a. *Long-Term Adherence:*
- Plant-based diets are often more sustainable and enjoyable for individuals, increasing the likelihood of long-term adherence to healthy eating habits.

b. Flexible and Varied Choices:
- The flexibility and variety within plant-based diets allow for a diverse range of culinary options, making it easier to maintain the lifestyle.

9. Support for Mental Health:

a. Nutrient-Rich Foods for Brain Health:
- Nutrient-dense plant foods provide essential vitamins and minerals that support overall brain health, potentially benefiting mental well-being.

b. Stress Reduction:
- The anti-inflammatory and stress-reducing properties of plant-based diets may positively impact mental health, which is crucial in diabetes management.

Conclusion:

A plant-based diet offers a multifaceted approach to managing Type 2 Diabetes, addressing various aspects of health, from blood sugar control to cardiovascular well-being. The numerous benefits make it a viable and sustainable lifestyle choice for individuals seeking to improve their overall health in the context of diabetes management.

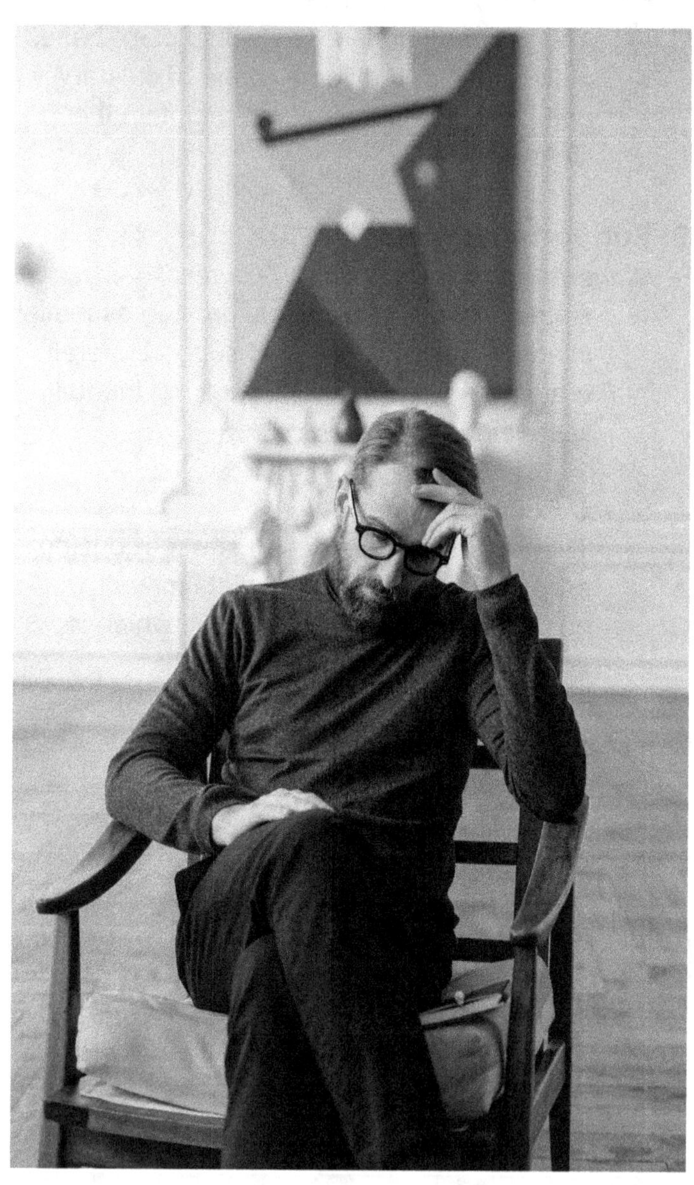

CHAPTER EIGHT

Improving Mental Health and Well-being

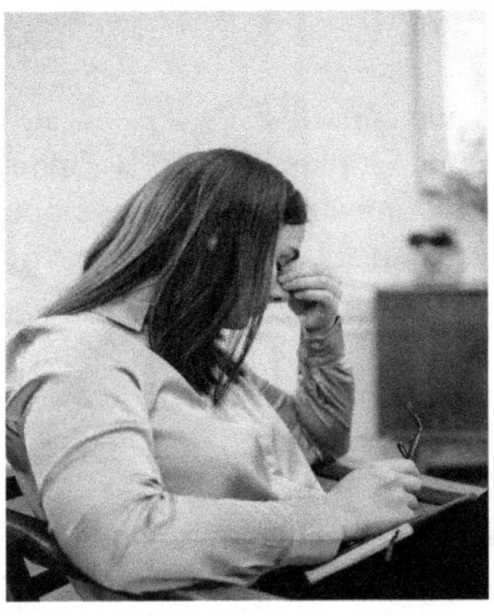

Mood and Cognitive Benefits

Adopting a plant-based diet not only positively impacts physical health but also contributes significantly to mood and cognitive well-being. Here's a detailed analysis of the numerous benefits associated with a plant-based lifestyle:

1. Nutrient-Rich Foods for Cognitive Function:

a. Antioxidants and Phytochemicals:
- Plant-based foods are rich in antioxidants and phytochemicals, which protect the brain from oxidative stress and support cognitive function.

b. Vitamins and Minerals:
- Essential nutrients like B-vitamins, folate, and magnesium found in plant-based foods play a crucial role in maintaining cognitive health and mental clarity.

2. Inflammation Reduction:

a. Anti-Inflammatory Properties:
- Plant-based diets are associated with lower levels of inflammation, reducing the risk of chronic diseases and promoting a healthy brain.

b. Omega-3 Fatty Acids:
- Incorporating plant-based sources of omega-3 fatty acids, such as flaxseeds and walnuts, helps combat inflammation and supports cognitive function.

3. Gut-Brain Connection:

a. Healthy Gut Microbiome:

- The fiber-rich content of plant-based diets fosters a healthy gut microbiome, positively influencing mood and cognitive health through the gut-brain axis.

b. Probiotic-Rich Foods:

- Fermented plant-based foods contribute to a balanced gut microbiota, potentially enhancing mental well-being.

4. Blood Sugar Regulation:

a. Stable Blood Sugar Levels:

- Plant-based diets, rich in fiber, help stabilize blood sugar levels, preventing energy crashes and mood swings associated with blood sugar fluctuations.

b. Reduced Risk of Type 2 Diabetes:

- By promoting weight management and insulin sensitivity, plant-based diets reduce the risk of Type 2 Diabetes, a condition linked to cognitive decline.

5. Serotonin Production and Mood Enhancement:

a. Tryptophan-Rich Foods:
- Plant-based sources of tryptophan, like seeds and legumes, contribute to serotonin production, promoting a positive impact on mood.

b. Carbohydrates and Serotonin:
- The inclusion of whole, unprocessed carbohydrates in plant-based diets supports serotonin synthesis, contributing to overall mood enhancement.

6. Weight Management and Positive Body Image:

a. Maintaining a Healthy Weight:
- Plant-based diets are often associated with weight management, positively influencing body image and contributing to improved mood.

b. Enhanced Self-Esteem:
- Achieving and maintaining a healthy weight through plant-based eating can boost self-esteem, positively impacting cognitive well-being.

7. Cardiovascular Health Benefits:

a. Cholesterol Reduction:
- The heart-healthy nature of plant-based diets contributes to better cardiovascular health, reducing the risk of conditions that could impact cognitive function.

b. Blood Pressure Control:
- Plant-based diets, rich in potassium from fruits and vegetables, support healthy blood pressure levels, positively influencing cognitive health.

8. Cognitive Reserve and Aging:

a. Neuroprotective Effects:
- The antioxidants and anti-inflammatory compounds found in plant-based foods may have neuroprotective effects, potentially reducing the risk of cognitive decline with age.

b. Building Cognitive Reserve:
- Engaging in a plant-based lifestyle may contribute to building cognitive reserve, enhancing the brain's ability to withstand age-related changes.

9. Improved Sleep Quality:

a. Magnesium-Rich Foods:

- Plant-based diets, rich in magnesium, contribute to improved sleep quality, positively impacting both mood and cognitive function.

b. Melatonin Precursors:

- Some plant foods, like tart cherries, contain precursors to melatonin, a hormone that regulates sleep-wake cycles.

10. Mindful Eating Practices:

a. Increased Mindfulness:

- The emphasis on whole, plant-based foods encourages mindful eating practices, fostering a positive relationship with food and reducing stress.

b. Mind-Gut Connection:

- Mindful eating may positively impact the mind-gut connection, influencing mood and cognitive function through the gut-brain axis.

Conclusion:

A plant-based diet's impact on mood and cognitive function is multifaceted, encompassing nutrient-rich foods, anti-inflammatory properties, and support for gut health. By embracing a plant-based lifestyle, individuals can enhance both their physical and mental well-being, contributing to a holistic approach to health.

Impact on Mental Health Conditions

Adopting a plant-based diet can have profound effects on mental health, positively influencing various conditions. Here's a detailed analysis of the impact of plant-based diets on mental well-being:

1. Depression and Anxiety:
a. Nutrient-Rich Foods:
- Plant-based diets, rich in vitamins, minerals, and antioxidants, provide essential nutrients that support brain health, potentially alleviating symptoms of depression and anxiety.

b. Omega-3 Fatty Acids:
- Including plant-based sources of omega-3 fatty acids, like flaxseeds and chia seeds, may have mood-stabilizing effects.

2. Stress Reduction:
a. Complex Carbohydrates:
- Whole, unprocessed carbohydrates found in plant-based diets contribute to the production of serotonin, a neurotransmitter that helps regulate mood and reduce stress.

b. Adaptogenic Herbs:
- Some plant-based foods, such as adaptogenic herbs like ashwagandha and holy basil, may assist in reducing stress levels.

3. Cognitive Function and Focus:

a. Antioxidant-Rich Foods:

- Plant-based diets, abundant in fruits and vegetables, provide antioxidants that protect the brain from oxidative stress, supporting cognitive function and focus.

b. Low-Glycemic Foods:

- Emphasizing low-glycemic index foods helps maintain steady blood sugar levels, preventing energy crashes that can affect concentration.

4. ADHD and Hyperactivity:

a. Elimination of Food Additives:

- Plant-based diets often exclude artificial additives and preservatives that may exacerbate symptoms of ADHD and hyperactivity.

b. Balanced Nutrient Intake:

- Ensuring a well-balanced intake of nutrients supports overall brain health, potentially influencing ADHD symptoms.

5. Bipolar Disorder:

a. Stable Blood Sugar Levels:

- Plant-based diets, with their emphasis on fiber and complex carbohydrates, contribute to stable blood sugar levels, which may have a positive impact on mood stability.

b. *Omega-3 Fatty Acids:*
- Plant-based sources of omega-3 fatty acids may play a role in mood regulation, potentially benefiting individuals with bipolar disorder.

6. Sleep Disorders:
a. *Melatonin-Rich Foods:*
- Some plant-based foods, like tart cherries and tomatoes, contain melatonin precursors that may aid in regulating sleep-wake cycles.

b. *Magnesium-Rich Foods:*
- Plant-based diets, rich in magnesium from leafy greens and nuts, contribute to improved sleep quality.

7. Eating Disorders:
a. *Focus on Whole Foods:*
- A plant-based diet that emphasizes whole, nutrient-dense foods may promote a healthier relationship with food, potentially benefiting those recovering from eating disorders.

b. *Supportive Nutrient Intake:*
- Ensuring an adequate intake of essential nutrients supports overall physical and mental health during the recovery process.

8. Schizophrenia and Psychosis:

a. Anti-Inflammatory Effects:
- Plant-based diets, with their anti-inflammatory properties, may have potential benefits for individuals with schizophrenia, as inflammation is implicated in the disorder.

b. Balanced Nutrient Intake:
- Ensuring a balanced intake of essential nutrients supports overall brain health and may play a role in managing symptoms.

9. Social Connection and Community:

a. Engagement in Plant-Based Communities:
- Joining plant-based communities fosters a sense of belonging and social connection, contributing to mental well-being.

b. Shared Lifestyle Choices:
- Sharing a plant-based lifestyle with others can create a supportive environment that positively impacts mental health.

10. Overall Well-Being:

a. Positive Impact on Lifestyle:
- Adopting a plant-based diet often encourages other positive lifestyle choices, such as regular physical activity and mindfulness practices, contributing to overall well-being.

b. Ethical Considerations
- Aligning dietary choices with ethical considerations, such as environmental sustainability and animal welfare, may positively impact mental well-being.

Conclusion:

While adopting a plant-based diet may not replace professional mental health interventions, it can play a supportive role in promoting overall well-being. Nutrient-rich plant foods, anti-inflammatory effects, and a focus on whole, unprocessed ingredients contribute to a holistic approach to mental health.

Part III: Practical Aspects and Resources

CHAPTER NINE

Recipes and Meal Plans

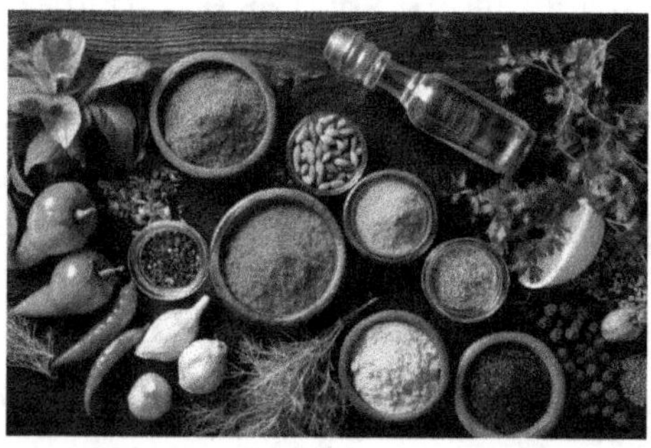

Nutrient-Dense Plant-Based Recipes

Nutrient-dense Plant-Based Recipes Packed with Essential Nutrients

1. **Almond Butter Energy Bites**
   - Quick and easy bites packed with dates, and chia seeds for a boost of energy.

2. **Avocado Pesto Zoodles**
   - Zucchini noodles tossed in a creamy avocado pesto sauce with cherry tomatoes and pine nuts.

3. **Almond Berry Smoothie Bowl**
   A delightful blend of almonds, mixed berries, and banana topped with granola and chia seeds.

4. **Avocado and Black Bean Salad**
   - A refreshing salad featuring creamy avocado, black beans, corn, cherry tomatoes, and lime dressing.

5. **Baked Falafel Wraps**
   - Crispy baked falafel wrapped in whole-grain tortillas with fresh veggies and tahini sauce.

6. **Banana Walnut Oat Pancakes**
   - Fluffy oat-based pancakes with ripe bananas and chopped walnuts, perfect for a wholesome breakfast.

7. **Black Bean and Corn Salsa**
   - A vibrant salsa featuring black beans, corn, red onion, cilantro, and lime juice, ideal as a topping or dip.

8. **Blueberry Spinach Smoothie**
   - A refreshing smoothie blend of
     blueberries, spinach, banana, and
     almond milk for a nutrient-packed
     start to the day.

9. **Broccoli and Chickpea Stir-Fry**
   - Quick stir-fry combining broccoli,
     chickpeas, and colorful bell peppers
     in a savory soy-ginger sauce.

10. **Baked Stuffed Bell Peppers**
    - Bell peppers filled with quinoa, black
      beans, corn, and spices, baked to
      perfection.

11. **Cauliflower Buffalo Wings**
    - Baked cauliflower florets coated in
      spicy buffalo sauce for a healthier
      take on classic buffalo wings.

12. **Chia Seed Pudding Parfait**
    - Layered chia seed pudding with
      fresh fruit, granola, and a drizzle of
      maple syrup for a delightful dessert
      or breakfast.

13. **Coconut Quinoa Curry**
    - A rich and flavorful curry with
      quinoa, coconut milk, chickpeas, and
      a blend of aromatic spices.

14. Crispy Baked Sweet Potato Fries

- Oven-baked sweet potato fries seasoned with paprika and garlic, served with a tangy dipping sauce.

15. Cucumber Avocado Rolls

- Refreshing cucumber rolls filled with creamy avocado, radishes, and sprouts, perfect for a light snack.

16. Cauliflower and Chickpea Curry

- A flavorful curry with cauliflower, chickpeas, and a blend of aromatic spices served over brown rice.

17. Chia Seed Breakfast Pudding

- Chia seeds soaked in almond milk with vanilla extract, topped with fresh fruit and nuts.

18. Coconut Lentil Soup

- A hearty soup made with lentils, coconut milk, and a mix of vegetables for a nourishing meal.

19. Dark Chocolate Avocado Mousse

- Silky chocolate mousse made with ripe avocados, dark cocoa, and a touch of maple syrup.

20. Eggplant and Tomato Stacks

- Sliced eggplant and tomato stacks baked with herbs and a balsamic glaze.

21. Farro and Vegetable Buddha Bowl

- A wholesome Buddha bowl featuring farro, roasted vegetables, and a tahini dressing.

22. Green Goddess Quinoa Bowl

- Quinoa bowl with a variety of green vegetables, avocado, and a herb-infused dressing.

23. Kale and Pomegranate Salad

- Nutrient-packed salad featuring kale, pomegranate seeds, walnuts, and a citrusy vinaigrette.

24. Mango Salsa Stuffed Sweet Potatoes

- Baked sweet potatoes filled with vibrant mango salsa, black beans, and cilantro.

25. Mushroom and Spinach Stuffed Portobellos

- Portobello mushrooms stuffed with a savory mixture of sautéed mushrooms, spinach, and breadcrumbs.

26. Quinoa and Vegetable Stir-Fry

- Quinoa stir-fried with a colorful medley of vegetables in a soy-ginger sauce.

27. Rainbow Power Salad

- Use a variety of leafy greens like spinach, kale, and arugula as the base. Add chopped vegetables like bell peppers, cherry tomatoes and cucumber.

28. Spaghetti Squash Primavera

- Roasted spaghetti squash tossed with a medley of fresh, sautéed vegetables in a light tomato sauce.

29. Sweet Potato and Kale Hash

- A hearty breakfast hash featuring sweet potatoes, kale, and a sprinkle of nutritional yeast.30.

30. Tomato Basil Zucchini Noodles

- Zucchini noodles tossed in a flavorful tomato and basil sauce, topped with pine nuts.

31. Turmeric Chickpea Stew

- A warming stew with chickpeas, turmeric, and a mix of vegetables for a comforting, immune-boosting dish.

32. Vegan Caesar Salad

- A plant-based twist on the classic Caesar salad with crisp romaine lettuce, vegan Caesar dressing, and croutons.

33. Walnut Pesto Pasta

- Whole-grain pasta coated in a rich walnut pesto sauce, complemented by cherry tomatoes and arugula.

34. Yellow Split Pea Dal

- Dal made with yellow split peas, spices, and tomatoes, served over brown rice for a protein-packed meal.

35. Zesty Lemon Asparagus Quinoa

- Quinoa mixed with sautéed asparagus, lemon zest, and fresh herbs for a light and flavorful side dish.

Plant- based diet Weekly Meal Plans

FOR WEEKS ONE AND TWO

SUNDAY

BREAKFAST
- Acai bowl topped with granola, coconut flakes, and mixed berries.

LAUNCH
- Chickpea salad sandwich on whole grain bread with lettuce and tomatoes.

DINNER
- Rice cakes topped with almond butter and sliced banana

SATURDAY

BREAKFAST
- Vegan French toast made with plant-based milk and cinnamon, topped with fresh berries and maple syrup.

LAUNCH
- Falafel wrap with tahini sauce, lettuce, cucumbers, and tomatoes.

DINNER
- Vegetable stir-fried noodles with tofu or tempeh.

MONDAY

BREAKFAST

- Overnight oats topped with mixed berries and almond butter.

LAUNCH

- Quinoa salad with roasted vegetables (such as bell peppers, zucchini, and eggplant) and a lemon-tahini dressing.

DINNER

- Lentil curry with brown rice and a side of steamed broccoli.

TUESDAY

BREAKFAST

- Smoothie made with almond milk, spinach, banana, and a scoop of plant-based protein powder.

LAUNCH

- Whole grain wrap filled with hummus, roasted vegetables, and mixed greens.

DINNER

- Chickpea and vegetable stir-fry with quinoa.

WEDNESDAY

BREAKFAST

Avocado toast on whole grain bread sprinkled with nutritional yeast and a side of sliced tomatoes.

LAUNCH

Mixed greens salad with cherry tomatoes, cucumbers, chickpeas, and a light vinaigrette dressing.

DINNER

Vegan chili with beans, tomatoes, bell peppers, and spices.

THURSDAY

BREAKFAST
- Tofu scramble with sautéed mushrooms, spinach, and onions, served with whole grain toast.

LAUNCH
- Mediterranean quinoa salad with diced tomatoes, cucumber, olives, red onion, and a lemon-herb dressing.

DINNER
- Sweet potato and black bean enchiladas with a side of roasted Brussels sprouts.

FRIDAY

BREAKFAST
- Vegan protein pancakes with a side of fresh fruit.

LAUNCH
- Curry lentil soup with a side of whole grain bread.

DINNER

Quinoa-stuffed bell peppers with a side of steamed asparagus.

FOR WEEKS 3 AND 4
SUNDAY

BREAKFAST- Avocado Toast with Cherry Tomatoes

LAUNCH - Quinoa Salad with Chickpeas, Cucumbers, and Lemon-Tahini Dressing

DINNER - Lentil and Vegetable Stir-Fry with Brown Rice

SATURDAY

BREAKFAST - Berry Smoothie Bowl with Almond Butter and Granola

LAUNCH - Spinach and Chickpea Salad with Balsamic Vinaigrette

DINNER - Sweet Potato and Black Bean Enchiladas

MONDAY

BREAKFAST - Oatmeal with Sliced Bananas and Walnuts

LAUNCH - Mediterranean Wrap with Hummus, Olives, and Fresh Vegetables

DINNER- Roasted Cauliflower and Chickpea Curry with Quinoa

TUESDAY

BREAKFAST - Chia Seed Pudding with Mixed Berries

LAUNCH - Stuffed Bell Peppers with Quinoa and Black Beans

DINNER- Zucchini Noodles with Tomato-Basil Sauce

<h1 style="text-align:center">WEDNESDAY</h1>

BREAKFAST

- Green Smoothie with Kale, Pineapple, and Coconut Water

LAUNCH

- Lentil and Vegetable Soup with Whole Grain Bread

DINNER

- Teriyaki Tofu Stir-Fry with Brown Rice

<h1 style="text-align:center">THURSDAY</h1>

BREAKFAST

- Whole Grain Pancakes with Maple Syrup and Fresh Fruit

LAUNCH

- Greek Salad with Tofu Feta and Kalamata Olives

DINNER

- Eggplant and Tomato Stacks with Balsamic Glaze

<h1 style="text-align:center">FRIDAY</h1>

BREAKFAST

- Vegan Breakfast Burrito with Black Beans and Avocado

LAUNCH

- Quinoa-Stuffed Portobello Mushrooms

DINNER

- Coconut Lentil Soup with Sliced Baguette

CHAPTER TEN

Shopping Guide for Plant-Based Eating.

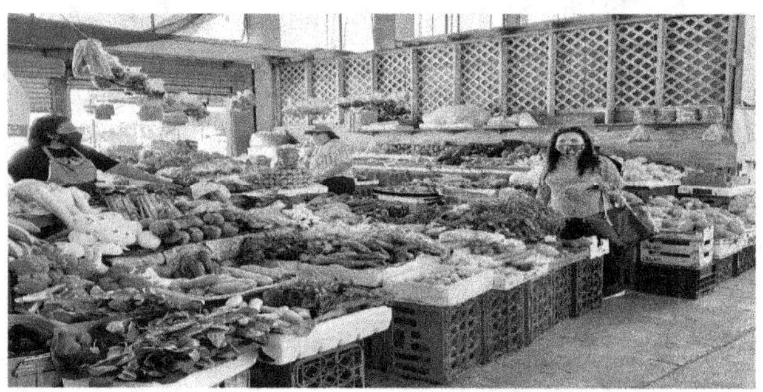

Selecting Fresh Produce

Shopping for fresh produce is an essential part of plant-based eating.. By choosing high-quality fruits and vegetables, you can ensure you're getting a wide range of nutrients and flavors in your plant-based meals.

Plan your meals:

Before heading to the grocery store or farmer's market, plan your meals for the week leveraging on the Plant-based diet weekly meal plan as prepared in Chapter 9 above. This will help you determine what types of produce you need and in what quantity. Here is a detailed shopping guide to help you select the best fresh produce for your plant-based diet

1. Vegetables:

- Leafy greens: Look for vibrant, crisp, and unwilted leaves. Avoid any with discoloration or slimy patches.

- Cruciferous vegetables (broccoli, cauliflower, Brussels sprouts): Choose firm heads with compact florets. Avoid any with soft spots or yellowing.

- Root vegetables (carrots, beets, radishes): Select vegetables that are firm and free from blemishes. Avoid any that are soft or have moldy patches.

- Tomatoes: Opt for tomatoes that have bright red or vibrant colors, depending on the variety. They should feel firm but yield slightly to gentle pressure.

- Peppers: Choose peppers that are firm, glossy, and have taut skin. Avoid any with wrinkles or soft spots.

2. Fruits:

- Citrus fruits: Look for fruits that feel heavy for their size, indicating juiciness. Avoid any with soft spots or mold.

- Berries: Select berries that are plump, brightly colored, and free from mold or mushy spots.
- Apples: Choose apples that are firm, smooth, and have vibrant colors. Avoid any with bruises or shriveled skin.
- Bananas: Select bananas based on your preferred ripeness. Green bananas will take longer to ripen, while yellow bananas are ideal for immediate consumption.
- Stone fruits (peaches, plums, nectarines): Choose fruits that are slightly soft to the touch, indicating ripeness. Avoid any with bruises or overly wrinkled skin.

3. Herbs:

- Look for fresh herbs that are vibrant in color, aromatic, and have no signs of wilting or discoloration.
- Avoid herbs with yellowed or brown leaves, as these are indications of aging and loss of flavor.

4. Buying in-season produce:

- Purchasing fruits and vegetables that are in-season ensures better flavor, quality, and usually more affordable prices.
- Familiarize yourself with the seasonal produce in your region and purchase accordingly.

5. Organic produce:

- Organic options are free from synthetic fertilizers, pesticides, and genetic modifications.
- Choose organic produce, especially for items on the "Dirty Dozen" list, which includes produce with higher pesticide residues.

3. Farmer's markets:

Whenever possible, consider shopping at farmer's markets. Locally grown produce typically has a shorter time between harvest and sale, resulting in fresher and more nutritious produce. Additionally, talking to the farmers gives you an opportunity to learn about different varieties and cooking methods.

4. Freshness indicators:

While shopping, keep an eye out for freshness indicators to ensure you're selecting the best produce. Here are some tips for selecting the best quality fruits and vegetables:

★ **Appearance:**
Choose produce that has bright, vibrant colors, as they are usually a good indication of freshness and nutrient content. Avoid fruits and vegetables that appear dull or have blemishes.

★ **Texture:**
The texture of produce can give you a clue about its freshness. For example, soft or mushy fruits may have started to spoil, while crisp and firm vegetables are usually fresher. Check for firmness or crispness. Some vegetables, like cucumbers or bell peppers, should feel firm and taut, while others, like tomatoes or avocados, should have a slight give.

★ **Smell:**
Some fruits and vegetables, like melons or herbs, should have a pleasant aroma. However, others, like onions or garlic, may have a stronger odor. Trust your senses and avoid any produce with foul or moldy smells.Give the fruits and vegetables a gentle sniff. A pleasant and fresh aroma is a sign of good quality. If there is an unpleasant odor or no aroma at all, it may indicate that the produce is not at its best.

★ **Check for bruises or mold:**
Inspect the produce carefully for any bruises, cuts, or mold. These can be indicators of spoilage. Avoid fruits and vegetables with these signs, as they are likely to deteriorate quickly.

5. Make use of the whole plant:
Don't forget to explore the entire plant. Many parts of the plant, such as beet greens, carrot tops, or broccoli stems, are edible and can be incorporated into your meals. This helps reduce food waste and maximizes the nutritional value of your produce.

6. Handling and Storing Fresh Produce:

To prolong the lifespan of your fresh produce and maintain its quality, follow these handling and storage recommendations:

Handle with care:
- Handle fruits and vegetables gently to avoid bruising or damaging them.

Wash before use:
- Rinse fruits and vegetables under running water before eating or cooking them. Use a vegetable brush to scrub the produce with firm skin like potatoes or cucumbers. This helps remove any dirt, bacteria, or pesticide residue.

Store properly:
- Different fruits and vegetables have different storage requirements. Some general tips include:

- Store leafy greens and herbs in a damp cloth or in airtight containers in the refrigerator.
- Keep fruits that produce ethylene gas, such as apples and bananas, separate from ethylene-sensitive vegetables like lettuce and broccoli.

Essential Pantry Items

Essential pantry items are the building blocks of a fully stocked kitchen. They consist of versatile ingredients that can be used in a wide range of recipes and provide the foundation for many meals. Here is a detailed list of essential pantry items:

1. **Grains and Legumes:**
   - Rice (white, brown, or basmati)
   - Pasta (spaghetti, penne & macaroni)
   - Lentils (green, red, or black)
   - Chickpeas
   - Beans (black, kidney, cannellini)

2. **Canned Goods:**
   - Diced tomatoes
   - Tomato sauce
   - Tomato paste
   - Coconut milk
   - Tuna/Salmon
   - Chicken broth or vegetable broth

3. **Spices and Seasonings:**
    - Salt (kosher or sea salt)
    - Black pepper
    - Paprika (smoked and sweet)
    - Cumin
    - Chili powder
    - Garlic powder
    - Onion powder
  - Dried herbs (oregano, basil, thyme)
    - Dried chili flakes

4. **Baking Essentials:**
    - All-purpose flour
    - Whole wheat flour
    - Baking powder
    - Baking soda
    - Granulated sugar
    - Brown sugar
    - Vanilla extract
    - Cocoa powder
    - Yeast
    - Salt

5. **Oils and Vinegars:**
    - Olive oil
    - Vegetable oil
    - Balsamic vinegar
    - White vinegar
    - Apple cider vinegar
    - Rice vinegar

6. Condiments and Sauces:
   - Soy sauce or tamari
   - Worcestershire sauce
   - Ketchup
   - Mustard (Dijon and whole grain)
   - Mayonnaise
   - Hot sauce
   - Honey
   - Maple syrup

7. Nuts, Seeds, and Dried Fruits:
   - Almonds
   - Walnuts
   - Cashews
   - Sunflower seeds
   - Chia seeds
   - Flaxseed
   - Raisins
   - Dried cranberries

8. Alternative Dairy and Meat Substitutes- Meat substitutes like tofu, tempeh, seitan, and plant-based burgers or sausages provide options for those transitioning to a plant-based diet. Consider these as occasional treats rather than daily staples and choose brands with whole food ingredients whenever possible.

CHAPTER ELEVEN

Dining Out and Social Situations

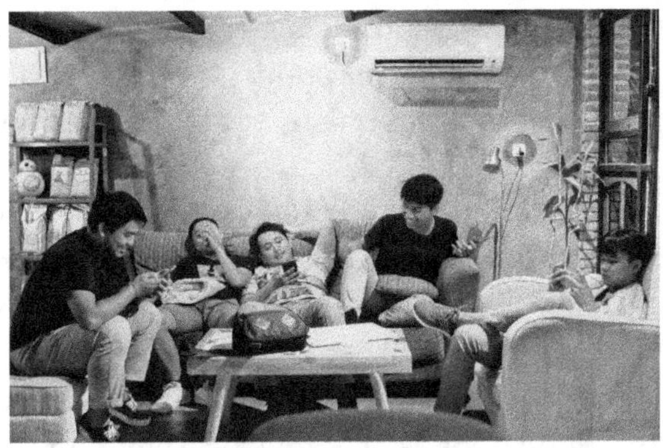

Navigating Restaurants and Events

Navigating restaurants and events as a plant-based diet can be an enjoyable experience with a bit of preparation and awareness. In this chapter, we shall be looking at some tips to make it easier:

1. Research in advance:

Before going to a restaurant or event, look up their menu or contact them to inquire about plant-based options. Many establishments nowadays provide plant-based or vegetarian/vegan choices but confirming beforehand can save you time and ensure there are suitable options available.

2. Ask for modifications:

If you find a dish on the menu that isn't entirely plant-based, don't hesitate to ask if they can modify it to meet your dietary preferences. Chefs are often willing to accommodate special requests.

3. Be specific with dietary requirements:

When ordering, clearly state that you follow a plant-based diet and request that no animal products, such as meat, fish, eggs, dairy, or honey, be included in your meal.

4. Look for vegetarian or vegan restaurants:

Seek out vegetarian or vegan restaurants in your area. These establishments are exclusively plant-based and offer a wider variety of options. Online directories or review platforms like HappyCow can help you find suitable restaurants.

5. Explore ethnic cuisines:

Many cultural cuisines have plant-based dishes as part of their traditional repertoire. Explore options like Indian, Middle Eastern, Thai, or Mexican restaurants, as these often have flavorful plant-based choices.

6. Be prepared with snacks:

In case you find yourself at an event or restaurant where plant-based options are limited, carry some snacks with you to keep yourself satiated. Nuts, seeds, fruit, or granola bars are portable options.

7. Communicate with event organizers:

If you're attending an event, such as a wedding or conference, inform the organizers in advance about your dietary requirements. This gives them the opportunity to plan plant-based options for you and other attendees.

8. Be flexible and creative:

If the available options aren't exactly what you were hoping for, consider being flexible and creative with your choices. Combine side dishes or request modifications to make a satisfying meal.

9. Connect with like-minded individuals:

Join local or online communities of people following a plant-based lifestyle. They can provide recommendations, share experiences, and offer suggestions for restaurants or events that cater well to plant-based diets.

10. Enjoy the experience:

Lastly, try to enjoy the dining or event experience while keeping in mind the positive contribution you are making to your health, the environment, and animal welfare. Focus on the tasty plant-based items.

Tips for Social Gatherings

Introduction:

Social gatherings can sometimes be challenging for individuals following a plant-based diet, especially when the majority of attendees consume animal products. However, with a little preparation and mindful decision-making, you can enjoy these events while staying true to your dietary choices. This chapter will provide you with practical tips and guidance to navigate social gatherings while adhering to a plant-based lifestyle.

1. **Communicate with the Host:**

Before attending a social gathering, it's a good idea to communicate with the host about your dietary preferences in a friendly and respectful manner. Let them know about your plant-based diet and offer to bring a plant-based dish to share. This can help create an inclusive atmosphere and ensure that there are options available for you.

2. **Offer to Help with the Menu:**

Suggest plant-based options that can be easily incorporated into the menu. Offer to provide ideas for plant-based appetizers, main dishes, or desserts. Sharing recipes or providing guidance on plant-based substitutes for traditional ingredients can be helpful for the host and increase the likelihood of having suitable options available.

3. **Plan and Prepare Ahead:**

If there are limited plant-based options available at the gathering, plan ahead and prepare your own dishes to bring along. Choose versatile and filling recipes, such as hearty salads, veggie skewers, or plant-based mains. Make sure to label your dish clearly to avoid any confusion.

4. **Be Mindful at the Buffet:**

If there's a buffet-style or self-serve setup, scout out the available options before diving in. Look for salad bars or veggie platters where you can create a well-rounded meal. Select dishes that are likely to be plant-based or can be easily modified by omitting or switching ingredients. Don't hesitate to ask the waiter or host about the ingredients used in specific dishes.

5. **Bring Plant-Based Snacks:**

In addition to your main dish, bring some plant-based snacks to enjoy or share. This will ensure that you have something to munch on while socializing and provide an opportunity to introduce others to delicious plant-based foods. Think about bringing hummus with veggie sticks, fruit tray, roasted chickpeas, or plant-based dips and crackers.

6. **Educate and Inform:**

Social gatherings can be great opportunities to educate others about plant-based diets. If someone asks about your food choices, engage in a friendly conversation and explain your reasons for following a plant-based lifestyle. This can help dispel myths, promote understanding, and even inspire others to try plant-based options.However, remember to approach the conversation with respect and avoid being too pushy or judgmental.

7. **Be open-minded:**

Sometimes, the available options may not perfectly align with your plant-based preferences. However, approach these situations with an open mind and try to find the best alternatives possible. For example, you could ask for a salad without cheese and add extra veggies or request a vegan sauce or dressing.

8. **Focus on side dishes & accompaniments:**

Even if the main course at an event does not cater to plant-based eaters, there are often side dishes, appetizers, and accompaniments that can be plant-based. Load up on salads, steamed vegetables, fruit platters, bread, dips, and other plant-based options available.

9. **Make simple swaps:**

If non-plant-based dishes are being served, consider making simple swaps to modify them. For example, you can request a burger without the meat or cheese and replace it with a plant-based patty and vegan cheese.

10. **Be prepared for questions:**

Some people may be curious about your plant-based dietary choices. Be prepared to answer questions in a positive and informative manner. Share your reasons for adopting a plant-based diet, such as health, environmental, or ethical considerations, without imposing your views on others.

11. **Focus on the social aspect:**

Remember that social gatherings are meant for connecting with others, so focus on enjoying the company and engaging in conversations rather than solely on food. Participate in activities, games, or conversations that take the focus away from the food aspect of the gathering.

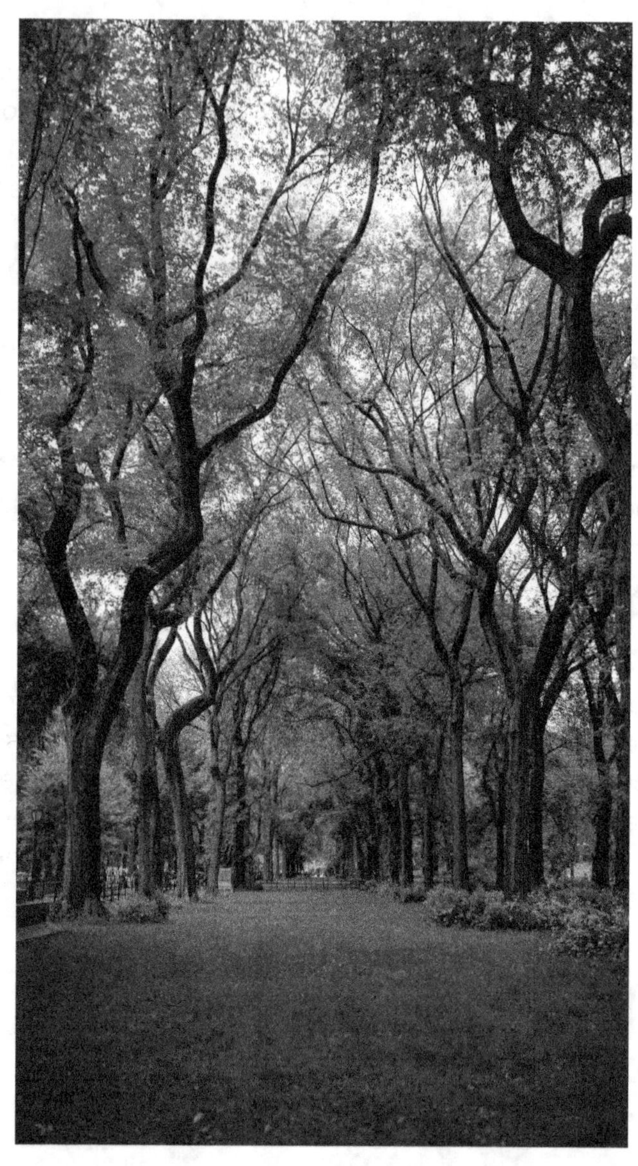

CHAPTER TWELVE

Sustainability and Environmental Impact

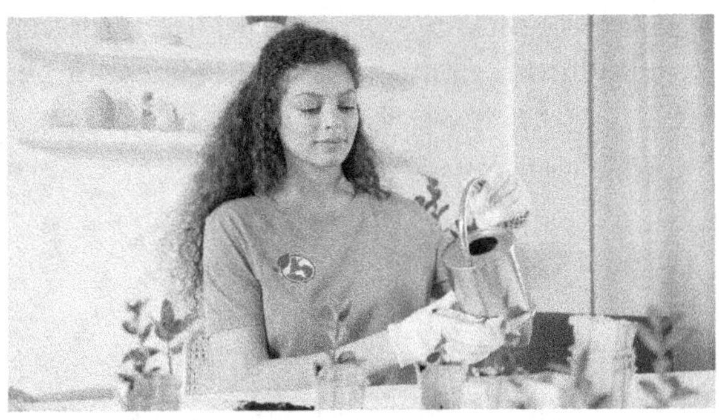

Environmental Impact of Plant-Based Diets

Introduction:

A plant-based diet, also known as a vegan or vegetarian diet, focuses on consuming foods derived from plants such as fruits, vegetables, grains, legumes, and nuts, while excluding or minimizing the intake of animal products. One of the most compelling reasons to adopt a plant-based diet is its positive impact on the environment. This comprehensive guide explores the environmental benefits of plant-based diets and sheds light on how our food choices can contribute to a more sustainable future.

1. **Reduced Greenhouse Gas Emissions:**
Animal agriculture is a frontline contributor to greenhouse gas emissions, particularly methane and nitrous oxide. These gases have a much higher warming potential than carbon dioxide.
The production, processing, and transportation of meat and animal products release substantial amounts of greenhouse gases into the atmosphere. Shifting towards plant-based diets reduces the demand for livestock, thereby mitigating greenhouse gas emissions and combating climate change.

2. **Conservation of Water Resources:**
Animal agriculture is incredibly water-intensive. Livestock farming requires vast quantities of water for drinking, irrigation, and the production of animal feed. By adopting a plant-based diet, individuals can significantly reduce their water footprint. Producing plant-based foods requires considerably less water compared to producing animal-based foods. Conserving water resources is crucial in mitigating water scarcity and preserving freshwater ecosystems.

3. **Preservation of Forests and Biodiversity:**
Animal agriculture is a leading driver of deforestation around the world. Forests are often cleared to make way for livestock grazing areas and to grow crops to feed farm animals. Deforestation not only contributes to climate

change but also results in the loss of valuable habitats and biodiversity. Conversely, plant-based diets require less land, allowing for the preservation of forests and protection of endangered species.

4. Mitigation of Land Degradation:

The expansion of animal agriculture often leads to land degradation through overgrazing, soil erosion, and nutrient depletion. In contrast, plant-based diets have the potential to reverse land degradation. By promoting sustainable farming practices like regenerative agriculture and organic farming, plant-based agriculture can enhance soil health, improve nutrient cycling, and restore degraded lands.

5. Reduced Pollution and Water Contamination:

The intensive use of fertilizers and pesticides in animal feed crops leads to water pollution, as these chemicals can leach into nearby water bodies. Furthermore, animal waste generated from large-scale factory farms often contaminates rivers, lakes, and groundwater. Adopting plant-based diets reduces the reliance on animal agriculture.

6. Reduction of water usage:

Animal agriculture is a major contributor to water scarcity. It takes a significant amount of water to raise livestock and grow feed crops. According to a study published in the journal Water Resources Research, producing one kilogram of beef requires an average of 15,415 liters of water, while producing one kilogram of vegetables requires only 322 liters. By adopting plant-based diets, we can reduce our water footprint and help conserve this precious resource.

7. Conservation of energy:

Animal agriculture is an inefficient process that requires a significant amount of energy inputs. From growing and transporting animal feed to running facilities and processing meat, there is a substantial energy expenditure associated with animal agriculture. In contrast, plant-based diets require fewer resources and less energy to produce. By shifting towards plant-based diets, we can conserve energy and reduce greenhouse gas emissions associated with the production of food.

8. Reduction of air pollution:

Animal agriculture is a significant source of air pollution. The production and transportation processes involved in raising livestock and processing animal products release various pollutants, including methane, ammonia, and nitrogen oxides. Livestock farming is estimated to be responsible for a significant proportion of global greenhouse gas emissions. Plant-based diets have a smaller carbon footprint and significantly reduce air pollution, contributing to improved air quality and mitigating climate change.

Contribution to Sustainability

The adoption of a plant-based diet contributes significantly to sustainability across various dimensions, including environmental, social, and economic aspects. Here's a detailed breakdown of how plant-based diets contribute to sustainability:

1. Environmental Impact:
Reduced Greenhouse Gas Emissions:
- Plant-based diets generally have a lower carbon footprint compared to animal-based diets.
- Livestock agriculture is a major contributor to greenhouse gas emissions, deforestation, and land degradation.

Conservation of Natural Resources:
- Plant-based diets require less land, water, and energy.
- Reduced reliance on animal farming helps conserve water resources and minimizes habitat destruction.

Mitigation of Deforestation:
- The expansion of agriculture, primarily for livestock, is a leading cause of deforestation.
- Plant-based diets alleviate the pressure on forests for grazing and feed production.

2. Biodiversity Conservation:

Preservation of Ecosystems:

- Plant-based diets contribute to the preservation of ecosystems and biodiversity.
- Reduced demand for animal products minimizes the negative impact on wildlife habitats.

Sustainable Agriculture Practices:

- Plant-based agriculture often aligns with more sustainable farming practices.
- Organic and regenerative farming methods support soil health and biodiversity.

3. Water Conservation:

Reduced Water Usage:

- Plant-based diets typically have a lower water footprint compared to animal-based diets.
- Livestock farming is water-intensive, contributing to water scarcity issues.

Efficient Water Allocation:

- Direct consumption of plant-based foods allows for more efficient water use in food production.
- Water is used directly for crop cultivation rather than being used for both crops and livestock.

4. **Social Impact:**

Equitable Resource Distribution:
- Plant-based agriculture can promote more equitable distribution of resources.
- Livestock farming often concentrates resources in certain regions, leading to inequitable access to land and water.

Food Security and Affordability:
- Plant-based diets can be more accessible and affordable for a broader population.
- Diversified plant foods offer a cost-effective and nutritious source of sustenance.

5. **Economic Sustainability:**

Diversification of Agriculture:
- Transitioning to plant-based agriculture encourages crop diversification.
- This diversification can enhance economic stability for farmers and communities.

Market Opportunities:
- The growing demand for plant-based products creates new market opportunities.
- Innovation in plant-based alternatives contributes to economic growth and job creation.

6. **Climate Change Mitigation:**

Mitigating Methane Emissions:

- Animal agriculture, particularly ruminant digestion, produces methane, a potent greenhouse gas.
- Plant-based diets contribute to mitigating methane emissions.

Promoting Sustainable Practices:

- Embracing plant-based diets encourages a shift toward sustainable agricultural practices.
- Sustainable farming methods contribute to climate change resilience.

7. **Global Health:**

Reduced Antibiotic Use:

- Plant-based diets are associated with a lower risk of zoonotic diseases, reducing the need for antibiotics in livestock.
- This contributes to the global effort to combat antibiotic resistance.

Improved Public Health:

- Plant-based diets are linked to numerous health benefits, reducing the burden on healthcare systems.
- A healthier population supports long-term social and economic sustainability.

Adopting and promoting plant-based diets aligns with broader sustainability goals, fostering environmental stewardship, social equity, and economic resilience. The collective shift towards plant-based eating plays a pivotal role in building a more sustainable and resilient future.

Conclusion

Summary of Benefits

A plant-based diet is a dietary approach that focuses primarily on foods derived from plants, such as fruits, vegetables, legumes, whole grains, nuts, and seeds, and limits or eliminates animal products. This type of diet offers several benefits for both our health and the environment. Here's a summary of the benefits of a plant-based diet:

1. **Improved heart health:**
Plant-based diets are associated with a reduced risk of heart disease, including lower blood pressure, decreased cholesterol levels, and a lower likelihood of developing cardiovascular conditions. This is because plant-based diets are typically low in saturated fat and rich in fiber, antioxidants, and heart-healthy nutrients.

2. **Weight management:**
Plant-based diets are generally lower in calories and higher in fiber compared to diets that include animal products.
These characteristics can contribute to weight management and reduce the risk of obesity. Additionally, plant-based diets are often more satiating, which can help control cravings and maintain a healthy weight.

3. **Lower risk of chronic diseases:** Plant-based diets have been linked to a lower risk of developing chronic conditions like type 2 diabetes, certain types of cancer (such as colon, breast, and prostate cancers), and other conditions such as metabolic syndrome and hypertension.

4. **Increased nutrient intake:**
Plant-based diets can provide a rich array of nutrients, including vitamins, minerals, antioxidants, and phytochemicals. Fruits, vegetables, whole grains, legumes, nuts, and seeds are abundant in essential nutrients such as folate, vitamin C, vitamin E, potassium, magnesium, and phytochemicals with potential health benefits.

5. **Improved digestion:**
Plant-based diets are typically high in dietary fiber, which promotes healthy digestion and prevents constipation. Whole grains, fruits, vegetables, and legumes provide a good amount of fiber, which supports a healthy gut microbiome and may reduce

the risk of conditions like diverticulitis and irritable bowel syndrome.

6. **Reduced risk of chronic diseases:** Plant-based diets have been associated with a lower risk of several chronic diseases. Studies have shown that individuals following a plant-based diet have a reduced risk of heart disease, high blood pressure, type 2 diabetes, certain types of cancer (such as colorectal and breast cancer), and obesity.

7. **Lower cholesterol levels:**
Animal products, particularly those high in saturated and trans fats, can raise cholesterol levels. In contrast, plant-based diets tend to be low in cholesterol and saturated fats and contain healthy fats, such as monounsaturated and polyunsaturated fats. This can help lower cholesterol levels and reduce the risk of heart disease.

8. **Environmental sustainability:** Plant-based diets have a smaller environmental footprint compared to diets that include animal products. The production of meat, especially from livestock, requires significant amounts of land, water, and energy. By opting for plant-based foods, individuals can help reduce greenhouse gas emissions, conserve water resources, and promote sustainable agricultural practices.

9. **Ethical considerations:**

Many people choose a plant-based diet due to ethical concerns about animal welfare. By avoiding or reducing the consumption of animal products, individuals can align their dietary choices with their values and support more humane treatment of animals.

10. **Increased variety and creativity in meals:**

Adopting a plant-based diet encourages individuals to explore a wider range of fruits, vegetables, whole grains, legumes, nuts, and seeds. This can lead to more diverse and exciting meals, as well as the opportunity to try new flavors and cooking techniques.

11. **Potential cost savings:**

Plant-based diets can be cost-effective, particularly when focusing on whole foods and seasonal produce. Staples like grains, beans, and legumes are usually more affordable than animal proteins, and planning meals around plant-based ingredients can help reduce overall food costs.

Remember that individual results and experiences may vary, and it's important to ensure you Consult with your dietician if it   becomes necessary to do so.

Encouragement for Sustaining a Plant-Based Life

Encouraging the sustenance of a plant-based lifestyle can be beneficial for both individuals and the environment. Here are some detailed strategies to promote and support plant-based living:

1. Education and Awareness:
- Provide comprehensive information on the benefits of a plant-based diet, including personal health benefits, environmental advantages, and ethical considerations.
- Offer workshops, seminars, and cooking classes to teach people about plant-based nutrition and how to prepare delicious plant-based meals.
- Share success stories and testimonials from individuals who have adopted a plant-based lifestyle to inspire others.

2. Accessibility and Affordability:
- Advocate for increased availability of plant-based food options in grocery stores, restaurants, and schools.
- Collaborate with local farmers' markets and community gardens to promote access to fresh, locally grown fruits and vegetables.
- Encourage government initiatives and subsidies that support plant-based

agriculture and make plant-based foods more affordable.

3. Health and Nutrition:

Work with healthcare professionals to provide accurate and up-to-date information on the health benefits of a plant-based lifestyle.

Develop partnerships with registered dietitians to offer personalized plant-based meal plans and guidance for individuals at various stages of their journey.

Organize health challenges or programs focused on giving participants the tools and resources to transition to and sustain a plant-based diet.

4. Culinary Innovation:

Promote culinary innovation by collaborating with chefs and restaurants to develop and showcase delicious plant-based dishes and menus.

Organize plant-based cooking competitions to highlight the creativity and diversity of plant-based cuisine.

Support food startups and entrepreneurs who are developing innovative plant-based alternatives to meat and dairy products.

5. Community and Support:

Establish local or online communities and support groups for individuals transitioning to or maintaining a plant-based lifestyle.

Organize social events, potlucks, or food festivals centered around plant-based cuisine, encouraging networking and sharing of experiences.

Provide mentorship or coaching programs to offer guidance and support for individuals seeking to adopt a plant-based lifestyle.

6. Environmental Advocacy:

Collaborate with environmental organizations to highlight the impact of animal agriculture and promote the adoption of plant-based diets as a solution to combat climate change.

Advocate for policies that promote sustainable farming practices and reduce the environmental footprint of the food system.

Support initiatives that encourage schools, hospitals, and other institutions to adopt plant-based menus and reduce their reliance on animal products.

Future of Plant-Based Eating

Introduction:
The future of plant-based eating presents a host of opportunities to transform our food systems, mitigate climate change, improve human health, and create a more sustainable and compassionate world.

I. Environmentally Sustainable Food Systems:
The rising demand for plant-based foods is directly correlated with the need for more environmentally sustainable food systems. Animal agriculture contributes significantly to greenhouse gas emissions, deforestation, and water pollution. In contrast, plant-based diets require fewer natural resources, emit fewer greenhouse gases, and have a lower ecological footprint. In the future, plant-based eating will play a crucial role in reducing our dependency on resource-intensive animal agriculture and transitioning to more sustainable food production systems.

II. Innovative Plant-Based Alternatives:
The future of plant-based eating will witness ongoing innovation and development of plant-based alternatives to animal-derived products. Advances in food technology and research have already led to a wide range of plant-based alternatives that closely mimic the taste, texture, and nutritional profile of traditional animal-based products. From plant-based meats,

cheeses, and dairy alternatives to egg substitutes and seafood alternatives, the market for plant-based foods is rapidly expanding. Continued innovation will ensure even more delicious and enticing plant-based options, appealing to a broader consumer base.

III. Health Benefits and Personal Wellness:

Plant-based diets have been associated with a myriad of health benefits. Increased consumption of fruits, vegetables, whole grains, legumes, and nuts can reduce the risk of chronic diseases, including heart disease, cancer, and diabetes. As the future of plant-based eating unfolds, more research and scientific insights will shed light on the specific health benefits and optimal dietary patterns. This knowledge will empower individuals to make informed choices regarding their personal wellness, leading to a shift towards plant-centric diets for health-conscious consumers.

IV. Mainstreaming of Plant-Based Eating:

The mainstream adoption of plant-based eating is well underway and will continue to expand in the coming years. Today, plant-based options are readily available in supermarkets, restaurants, and fast-food chains. As consumer demand for healthier, more sustainable food increases, businesses across the food industry are recognizing the economic opportunities.

V. Nutritional Impact of Plant-Based Eating

One of the key factors driving the future of plant-based eating is its positive nutritional impact. Plant-based diets have been associated with numerous health benefits. Such diets are typically rich in fiber, vitamins, minerals, and antioxidants, while being low in saturated fats and cholesterol. Consuming a variety of plant-based foods can help reduce the risk of chronic diseases like obesity, heart disease, type 2 diabetes, and certain types of cancer.

As the popularity of plant-based eating grows, there will be an increased emphasis on optimizing the nutritional value of plant-based foods. Researchers and food scientists will work to develop innovative ways to enhance the nutrient density and bioavailability of plant-based ingredients. This may involve techniques such as fortifying plant-based alternatives with essential vitamins and minerals, improving the absorption of nutrients through food processing methods, and developing new plant-based sources of key nutrients like omega-3 fatty acids and vitamin B12.

Furthermore, advancements in genetic engineering and biotechnology will play a role in developing new plant varieties with enhanced nutritional profiles. Scientists may be able to modify crops to be more nutrient-dense, resistant to pests and diseases, and adaptable to different environmental conditions. These advancements will contribute to the availability of a wider range of highly nutritious plant-based options, making it easier for individuals to meet their nutritional needs while following a plant-based diet.

Technological Innovations in Plant-Based Food

Technological innovations will continue to shape the future of plant-based eating. As consumer demand for plant-based alternatives increases, food companies will invest in research and development to create more advanced and realistic plant-based products.

One area of innovation lies in the development of plant-based meat alternatives. While the current generation of plant-based meats has made remarkable progress in terms of texture and taste, future innovations will likely focus on enhancing these attributes even further. Improvements in food science, biotechnology, and cellular agriculture will allow for the creation of plant-based meats that closely mimic the texture, juiciness, and flavor of animal-based meats. This will not only appeal to individuals seeking to reduce their meat consumption but also cater to meat lovers who are looking for sustainable and ethical alternatives.

Hope you got value from this guide book.
I will be glad you did.